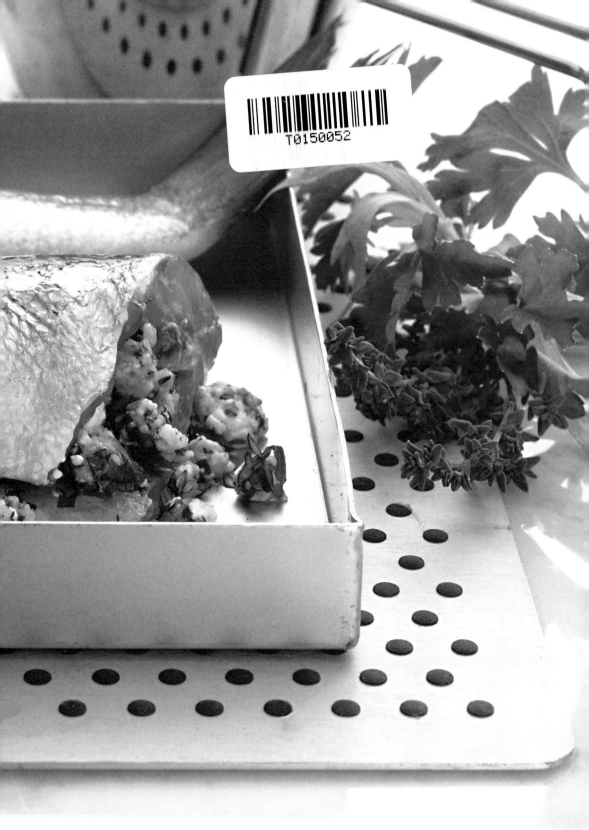

T0150052

THE LOW-FODMAP DIET

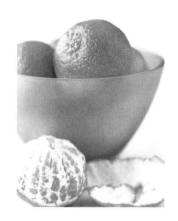

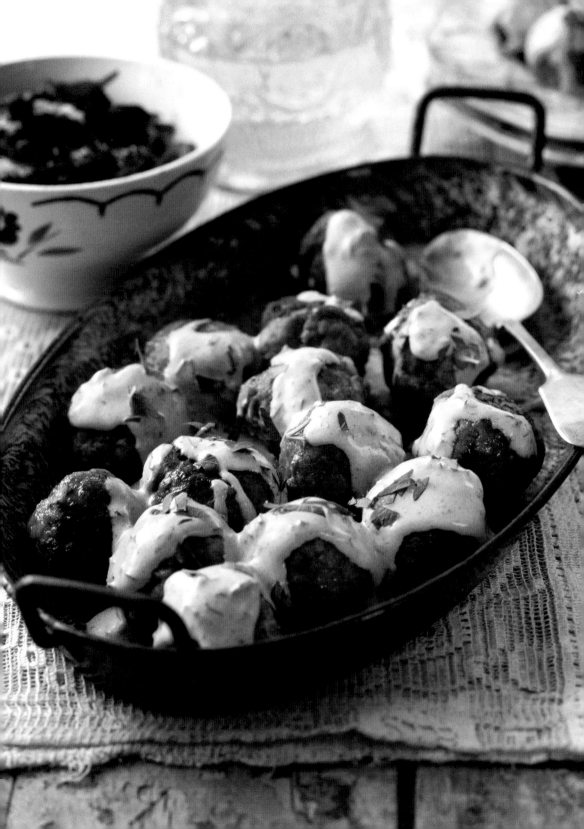

THE LOW-FODMAP DIET

AN EATING PLAN AND COOKBOOK

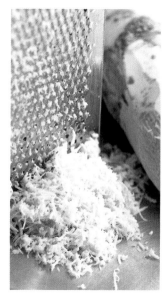
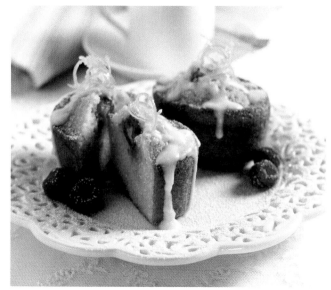

PENNY DOYLE

LORENZ BOOKS

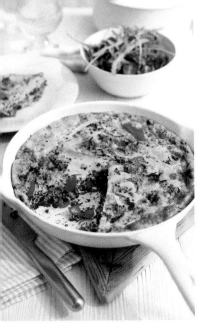
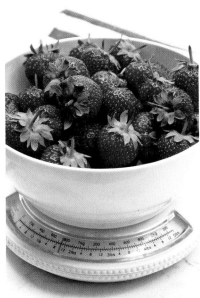
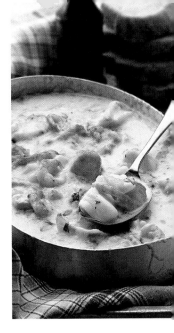

CONTENTS

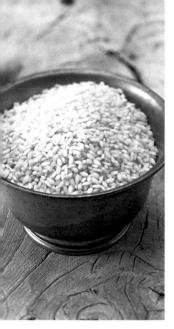
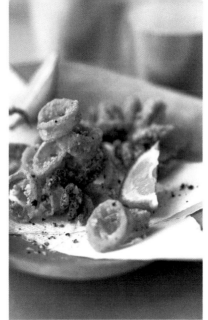
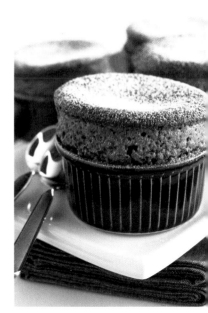

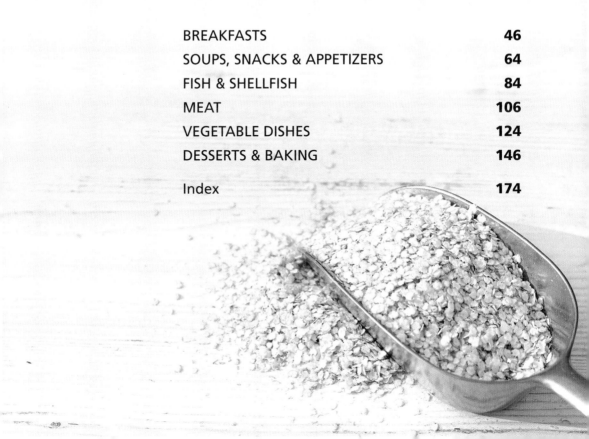

INTRODUCTION

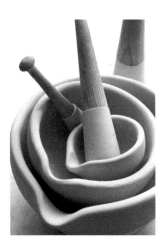

Irritable Bowel Syndrome (IBS) is a gut disorder that can considerably reduce an individual's quality of life, and affects up to a quarter of the population in developed countries. Symptoms are wide and varied, but commonly include diarrhoea, constipation, bloating and stomach pain. Since the 1950s the causes have been poorly understood, and treatment – based around changes in diet, medication and lifestyle – has always been challenging. In my work as a dietitian I have advised patients on treatment strategies that are based on national guidelines, but success has been limited. Exciting new research from Australia, however, has finally given hope to thousands of worldwide sufferers by examining the more precise links between IBS and diet, and we are able to advise sufferers more confidently with positive, measureable success.

FODMAP is an acronym for different types of carbohydrate foods that may contribute to IBS symptoms. Following a low-FODMAP diet is an elimination regime, which initially cuts out all potentially troublesome foods to find out if it improves your symptoms. This is followed by a controlled period of re-introduction of foods with the aim of establishing tolerances, and ideally increasing the range of foods that you can eat. You may initially feel that following a low-FODMAP diet takes considerable commitment. However, with this book to help you, and our detailed table of foods, you will quickly be able to see if the regime will help your condition.

In my practice I am seeing marked improvement of symptoms in around 70% of my IBS patients who try a low-FODMAP diet, with a significant increase in their quality of life. For some this can be profound, especially for those whose lives were dominated by their bowel habits, while others may simply feel less bloated and be more energetic. To support my clinical practice I am always looking for practical resources to support my patients, particularly where theory and recipe ideas are combined. My aim in this book is to use my wide experience to support you through your low-FODMAP trial and re-introduction. Armed with greater knowledge about managing symptoms though diet, your life could be transformed. The wide variety of dishes are full of flavour and goodness, with plenty of ideas for all types of meals, from breakfasts to entertaining, which I am confident will lift your spirits and keep your body comfortable!

PENNY DOYLE, Registered Dietitian

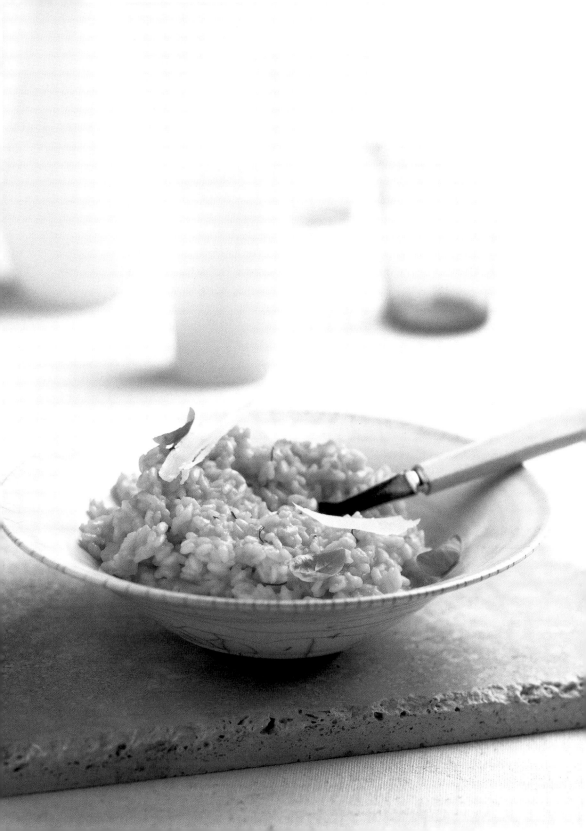

FODMAP FOOD TABLE

Use the table below as a quick and easy reference source for foods to avoid, limit or eat without restriction. When in the elimination phase of your low-FODMAP diet you should be rigorous about avoiding anything in the red column.

FOODS TO AVOID	RESTRICTED FOODS	GOOD TO EAT
These foods contain significant amounts of FODMAPs and should be avoided totally	These foods contain some FODMAPs and can be included in smaller amounts as indicated	These foods are free of FODMAPs and can be eaten freely
VEGETABLES AND PULSES	**VEGETABLES AND PULSES**	**VEGETABLES AND PULSES**
Asparagus	Artichoke hearts, no more than 2	Alfalfa
Baked beans	Avocado, no more than ¼ fruit	Aubergine (eggplant)
Black eyed peas (beans)	Beetroot (beet), no more than 4 slices	Bamboo shoots, beansprouts
Broad (fava) beans	Broccoli, chopped, no more than 45ml/3 tbsp	Cabbage, white
Butter (lima) beans	Brussels sprouts, fewer than 5	Capers
Cauliflower	Butternut squash, chopped, no more than 45ml/3 tbsp	Carrots
Chicory root	Celery, less than 5cm/2in of stick	Cassava
Garlic	Corn, no more than 45ml/3 tbsp	Celeriac
Hummus	Fennel, no more than 40g/1½oz	Chestnuts, water chestnuts
Jerusalem artichoke	Lentils, canned only, 90g/3½oz/ ½ cup	Chillies, red or green
Karela (bitter gourd)	Mangetouts (snow peas), fewer than 5 pods	Chives
Kidney beans	Okra, no more than 6 pods	Courgette (zucchini)
Leeks	Peas, no more than 45ml/3 tbsp	Cucumber
Lentils, dried red or yellow and dried split peas	Savoy cabbage, no more than 45ml/3 tbsp	Endive
Mushrooms	Sweet potato, chopped, no more than 45ml/3 tbsp	Fennel
Onions/shallots	Tomato, no more than 1 medium or 4 cherry	Gherkins
Pulses (eg chickpeas, soy beans, haricot (navy) beans etc)	Tomatoes, canned, 100g/4oz	Green beans
Spring onion (scallions), white part	Tomato, sundried, 4 pieces/ 15g/½oz	Ginger
Sugar snap peas		Kale
		Lettuce, any type
		Olives
		Pak choi (bok choy)
		Parsley, parsnip, (bell) peppers, plantain, potato, pumpkin
		Radish, radicchio, rocket (arugula)
		Seaweed (nori), spinach, spring onion (scallion), green part only, Swiss chard
		Yam

FOODS TO AVOID

FRUIT

Apples, fresh or dried

Apricots, fresh or dried

Bananas, overripe/brown

Blackberries

Boysenberries

Canned fruit in apple/pear juice

Coconut water

Dates

Figs

Lychees

Mango

Nectarines

Peaches

Pears

Persimmon

Plums

Prunes

Watermelon

HERBS, SPICES AND FLAVOURINGS

Curry pastes containing garlic or onion

Dried garlic or onion

Harissa paste with garlic

Pesto with garlic

Stock (bouillon) cubes, powder or granules containing garlic or onion

Teryaki marinade containing garlic or onion

Tomato/vegetable purée (paste) containing onion or garlic

Worcestershire sauce

RESTRICTED FOODS

FRUIT

Avocado, no more than ¼

Bananas, 1 small firm; fewer than 10 dried chips

Cherries, no more than 3

Clementines, no more than 2

Coconut, dried or desiccated (dried unsweetened shredded), no more than 45ml/3 tbsp

Dried fruit, any, 15ml/1 tbsp (13g/½oz)

Grapefruit, ½ medium

Grapes, no more than 10

Juice of low-FODMAP fruits, 100ml/3½fl oz/scant ½ cup

Kiwi fruit, no more than 2

Lychees, no more than 5

Mandarins, no more than 2

Melon, honeydew, 75g/3oz

Pineapple, 75g/3oz

Pomegranate, ½ of small

HERBS, SPICES AND FLAVOURINGS

Balsamic vinegar, 15ml/1 tbsp

Curry powder, 5ml/1 tsp

Miso paste, 30ml/2 tbsp

Tamarind, 2.5ml/½ tsp

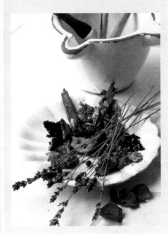

GOOD TO EAT

FRUIT

Blueberries

Breadfruit

Coconut, milk/cream/flesh

Cranberries (fresh)

Dragonfruit

Guava

Lemon, lime, including juice

Melon, canteloupe or galia

Orange

Passion fruit, papaya

Raspberries

Rhubarb

Satsumas

Strawberries

HERBS, SPICES AND FLAVOURINGS

Allspice, asofoetida

Basil

Capers, chilli powder/paste, chives, cinnamon, cloves, fresh or ground coriander (cilantro), cardamom

Egusi seeds

Fenugreek, fresh or dried, fish sauce (nam pla)

Garlic-infused oil (strained), ginger (fresh or dried), galangal

Horseradish sauce

Mustard (including seeds)

Nutmeg

Oyster sauce, olive oil and other vegetable oils

Parsley, pepper (black or white), poppy seeds (white)

Rosemary

Saffron, salt, shrimp paste, soy sauce, star anise, sundried tomato purée (onion and garlic-free)

Tabasco sauce, tahini paste, tarragon, thyme, turmeric

Vinegar (not balsamic)

Yeast extract

FOODS TO AVOID

PROTEINS

Any breaded meat or fish, as will contain wheat

Chorizo

Nuts, cashew and pistachio

Quorn products that contain wheat

CEREALS AND GRAINS

Barley

Chickpea (gram) flour

Couscous

Flavoured crisps (US potato chips) containing wheat

Gnocchi

Millet flour

Noodles made from wheat

Pea flour

Rye flour

Spelt bread (unless 100% sourdough)

Udon noodles

Wheat products where predominant ingredient is wheat flour: bread, pasta, cereals, cakes, biscuits, cookies

RESTRICTED FOODS

PROTEINS

Any processed meat or fish that might include wheat, for example sausage, salami, pâté, should be limited to a small portion

Nuts, almonds, no more than 10 whole or 100g/4oz ground; hazelnuts, no more than 10

CEREALS AND GRAINS

Amaranth, no more than 20g/¾oz/½ cup

Foods containing traces of wheat; stock (bouillon) cubes, thickened sauces

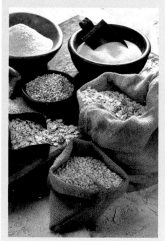

GOOD TO EAT

PROTEINS

All fish and seafood

All meat and game eg chicken, turkey, beef, ham, pork, duck, pheasant, venison

All seeds, eg pumpkin, sunflower, sesame, linseed

Eggs

Gelatine

Nuts: walnuts, peanuts, macadamia nuts, pine nuts

Quorn products, if wheat-free, soya protein/mince, tofu, tempeh

Sausages, if wheat-free and without onion or garlic

CEREALS AND GRAINS

Buckwheat flour, noodles and grain

Cornflakes, corn chips

Cornflour (cornstarch), cornmeal, maize, corn cakes

Crisps, plain

Oats/porridge, oatcakes

Polenta, popcorn

Quinoa

Rice cakes, rice noodles, rice (any type), puffed rice cereal

Sago, sourdough spelt bread, sorghum

Tapioca, teff

Wheat-free bread and 100% sourdough spelt bread

Xanthan gum

FOODS TO AVOID

CONDIMENTS, SUGARS, SWEETENERS AND SPREADS

Agave syrup, fructose, high fructose corn syrup (HFCS), Inulin, Isomalt, Maltitol, Mannitol, Sorbitol, Xylitol

Honey

Jam made with unsuitable fruits, marmalade/reduced-sugar jam containing polyols, check ingredients

Sugar-free sweets or chewing gum containing polyols, eg Sorbitol

Tomato ketchup, unless onion, garlic and wheat-free

DAIRY FOODS

Fromage frais

Low-fat Cheddar

Milk, buttermilk, evaporated milk, condensed milk

Processed cheese

Skimmed milk powder

Soya milk which uses 'whole' soya beans

Yogurt flavoured with unsuitable fruit, or honey, drinking or low-fat yogurt

DRINKS

Birch water (contains Xylitol)

Carbonated drinks (sodas) containing HFCS

Carob powder

Coconut water

Dessert wine

Herb teas such as fennel, apple, dandelion, chai, chamomile, and chicory drinks

Rum

Sports drinks containing Sorbitol/fructose

RESTRICTED FOODS

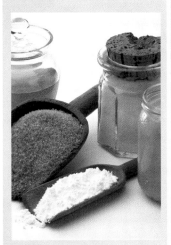

DAIRY FOODS

Cheese: cottage, cream cheese, low-fat soft, quark, less than 30ml/2 tbsp. Halloumi, less than 100g/4oz. Ricotta, less than 75g/3oz

Chocolate, any type, no more than 65g/2½oz

Custard, no more than 30ml/2 tbsp

Ice cream (1 scoop only)

Milk, cow/goat/sheep/A2, less than 45ml/3 tbsp

Yogurt flavoured with suitable fruit, less than 30ml/2 tbsp

DRINKS

Alcohol, spirits or wine, limit to 1–2 units a day

Beer, limit to 1 x 370ml/13fl oz/1½ cup bottle

Squash made using 'suitable' fruit for example orange, without added fructans such as HFCS, Sorbitol (see lists above)

Tea/coffee, limit to 2–3 cups a day

GOOD TO EAT

CONDIMENTS, SUGARS, SWEETENERS AND SPREADS

Aspartame (NutraSweet), Acesulfame K, Canderel, Dextrose, Hermesetas, Sucralose, Splenda, Saccharin

Jam made with suitable fruits

Marmalade without polyols, check ingredients

Sugar (sucrose) all, eg brown, white, molasses, maple syrup, palm sugar, treacle, stevia, golden (light corn) syrup

DAIRY FOODS

Any lactose-free or soya yogurt containing suitable fruits

Cheeses, all hard, full-fat, eg Cheddar, mozzarella, feta, brie, camembert, blue, Edam, any goat's

Cream, any type, crème fraîche, sour cream, butter, low-fat spread

Lactose-free/soya/oat/coconut/nut milks

Soya/lactose-free ice cream

DRINKS

Carbonated drinks without HFCS

Cocoa powder/drinking chocolate without lactose

Herb teas, peppermint or fruit teas not including 'unsuitable' fruit

UNTESTED FOODS

These foods have been used in our recipes, but at the time of writing the FODMAP content of them is unknown. They should be fine used in small quantities, but do consider excluding any of them that you think may be exacerbating your symptoms.

Black treacle	Juniper	Molasses	Sake
Cayenne	Kaffir lime leaves	Mooli (daikon)	Sage
Dashi no moto	Mint	Perilla/Shiso leaves	Yeast extract
Dill	Mirin	Pomegranate	

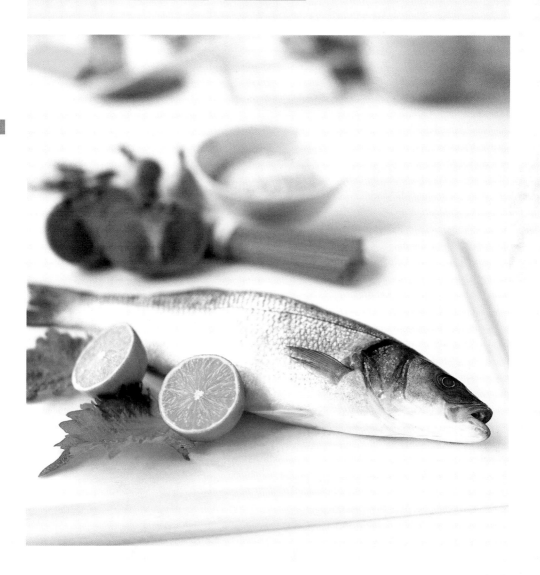

THE HUMAN DIGESTIVE TRACT

To help understand IBS, it is useful to know a little about the human digestive tract, which is effectively a long, closed tube that runs from the mouth to the anus, incorporating the mouth, oesophagus, stomach, small and large intestines.

UPPER DIGESTION

The purpose of the gut is to break down, or digest, food and pass nutrients to the blood for transportation around the body. Digestion occurs in many stages, starting with the action of saliva in the mouth and continuing in the stomach where food is temporarily stored and further broken down. Partially digested food then passes to the small intestine (ileum) where separate digestive enzymes work to break down individual food groups, for example fats, carbohydrates and proteins. The food then passes to the large intestine (colon) where different digestive enzymes get to work, processing broken-down nutrients, vitamins and minerals that the body can use. These partially digested nutrients are then passed through the gut wall into the blood for circulation. Carbohydrates are used as brain and muscle fuel, proteins for tissue growth and maintenance, and fats for cell structure and as an energy store. Fibre isn't broken down in the same way as other foods, as it serves mainly to help control the speed of digestion and maintain gut health.

LOWER DIGESTION

Little digestion occurs in the large intestine, or colon. The colon's main purpose is to reabsorb water, from food and drink, back into the body through its walls. There are also billions of bacteria in the gut, most of which are healthy, and some of which have an important role in digesting food by fermentation. This process also produces gases (mainly methane and hydrogen) that are harmless and are usually passed out as wind. If there is too much gas, or it becomes trapped, this can cause excessive bloating or flatulence, both of which are symptoms associated with IBS.

DISEASES OF THE DIGESTIVE TRACT

Various other problems can develop in the digestive tract, and to help you differentiate these from IBS, here are some of them.

IRRITABLE BOWEL SYNDROME (IBS)

IBS is considered a 'functional' disorder of the gut. The term 'functional' means that although the gut is still working well, there are unfortunate side effects in some people (see symptoms, page 16). IBS is not life-threatening, nor does it cause any adverse

This diagram shows the human digestive tract.

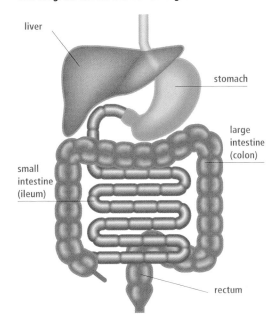

liver

stomach

large intestine (colon)

small intestine (ileum)

rectum

Introduction

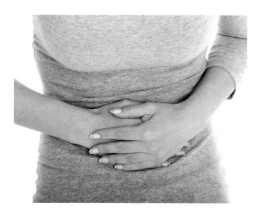

physical changes to the body, but it is a source of distress and anxiety for sufferers and their families. There is no specific test for IBS, it is diagnosed by a suitably qualified doctor who will consider the whole clinical picture.

COELIAC DISEASE (CD)
This disease is a reaction by the gut to gluten due to an inappropriate immune response. The body in effect 'over' reacts to the gluten found in wheat, rye and barley (and therefore in bread, baked goods, pasta etc), causing a range of gut and more general symptoms. It is hereditary, and unlike IBS, there are very specific clinical tests for its diagnosis. The only treatment is following a strict gluten-free diet. Unfortunately CD is often left undiagnosed for some years, particularly if symptoms, which are often the same as IBS, are mild. All IBS sufferers should be screened for CD.

Unfortunately some coeliacs may also suffer with IBS, and be symptomatic even after starting a gluten-free diet due to the presence of FODMAPs in the diet. Coeliacs wishing to trial the diet are likely to find many aspects easy as they will be accustomed to eating wheat-free alternatives to bread and carbohydrates. Although the low-FODMAP diet is wheat-free, some wheat-free foods may not also be gluten-free if contaminated during processing, so coeliacs need to be vigilant when checking suitable foods.

However, experience has proved that low-FODMAP, gluten-free diets are successful for some coeliacs with underlying IBS, and can help improve unpleasant gut problems such as bloating and looseness.

FOOD ALLERGY AND INTOLERANCES
True food allergy only affects up to 3% of the population, and symptoms can be potentially life-threatening if anaphylaxis (respiratory arrest) and heart failure result. Diagnosis using skin prick testing is clear-cut, but not widely available, and expensive. By comparison, food 'intolerance' is triggered by a different physiological mechanism, it can cause similar symptoms to allergy but is rarely life-threatening. These might include problems with the skin such as eczema, breathing difficulties like asthma, or gut problems, such as pain, bloating and looseness. Unfortunately tests using a finger-prick of blood, that are often available by post, are not reliable. Controlled elimination and the re-introduction of suspected foods, ideally with the help of a dietitian, is the most effective way to identify problem foods and ensure a balanced diet.

INFLAMMATORY BOWEL DISEASE (IBD)
This includes Crohn's disease, and Colitis, both of which are caused by an inappropriate inflammation of the gut, and for which there are very clear diagnostic markers. IBD can't be cured, but can be managed with medication and to some extent diet, though no particular food exclusion is required. Symptoms are similar to IBS, so it is important that IBS sufferers are screened to eliminate IBD.

CANCER
It is important to seek medical advice if there are any unexplained and regular changes in bowel habits. Cancers of the digestive tract can have similar symptoms to IBS, but with early detection are treatable, so do take the time to discuss the issues with your doctor.

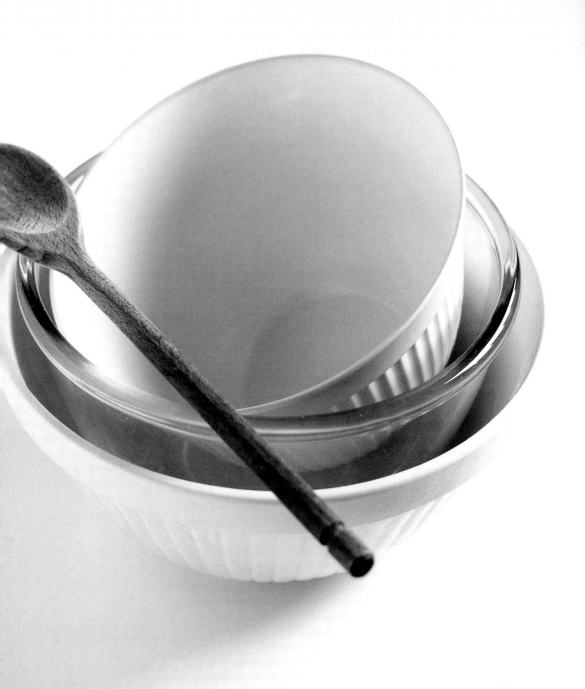

THE CAUSES OF IBS

There are several possible reasons for developing IBS, not all of them related to food and digestion. When you are considering trying the low-FODMAP diet you should address any of the other physiological, emotional and lifestyle causes of the disease so that you can also take action to tackle those.

STRESS AND EMOTIONS

Emotional factors are significant factors in the development of IBS, as the gut is made of smooth 'involuntary' muscle that is activated by stress hormones such as adrenaline. IBS sufferers tend to be generally more anxious about their health, often consider themselves to be medically more complex, and are more likely to consult their doctors regularly. In modern medicine it is now widely accepted that physiology (how the body works) and psychology (how the brain works) are very closely linked. Indeed a positive outlook and attitude can help combat many illnesses, including IBS. Some IBS sufferers may have a troubled past, including childhood abuse and psychiatric disorders, and may have emotional problems that impact on their everyday life. Studies have also shown that the bowels of people with IBS are more reactive to stress, and these individuals will experience more pain and looser stools than non-sufferers.

AGE AND GENDER

The incidence of IBS is higher in women, and also in younger people generally, so it is possible there may be a link with hormones. Genetics may of course also be an influence, though less is known about it.

PHYSIOLOGY

Other physical and biochemical factors are thought to contribute to IBS. One theory is that 'IBS' guts are more sensitive to pain, known as 'visceral hyperalgaesia'. So the abdominal discomfort or pain caused by

natural gases in the gut in an IBS sufferer may not be felt to the same degree by someone else. There may also be personal variations in the speed (known as 'motility') of the gut. Put simply an IBS sufferer with looser stools may just have faster-acting guts, so 'transit' of food happens more quickly. This may be the opposite for an IBS sufferer with firmer stools and constipation. If the gut works more slowly with a longer 'transit' time, it will lose more water along the way leading to firmer stools.

GUT BACTERIA

There has recently been more interest in the type and quantity of gut bacteria in IBS sufferers' guts. There is evidence that the number or type of these bacteria may be changed by past infections such as gastroenteritis or food poisoning, and

SYMPTOMS OF IBS

These vary in type and frequency between individuals, and may include some or all of the following:
• Diarrhoea and/or constipation
• Bloating and/or flatulence
• Abdominal pain
• Noisy gut ('borborygmus')
• Urgency (loss of control)
• 'Incomplete' evacuation (a feeling that the bowel has not properly emptied)
• Heartburn/reflux
• Nausea
• Lethargy (tiredness)

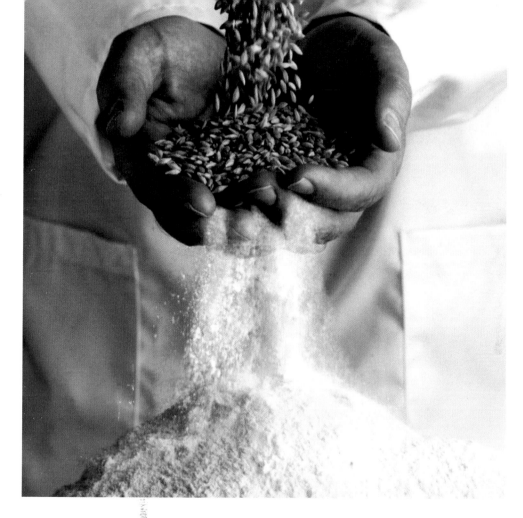

medications including antibiotics. If this is the case, then the type and amount of gases that the bacteria produce may change. Some bacteria are friendlier than others, and studies suggest that there are fewer 'good' bacteria, 'bifidobacter', in the guts of IBS sufferers. This is a fascinating science that warrants further research, and offers the potential of treatment that could focus on helping the gut to host more good bacteria.

FOOD AND DIET

The point of a low-FODMAP diet is to reduce the amount of potentially 'fermentable' foods in the large intestine that could cause bloating, wind, pain and diarrhoea. The

Many of our staple foods contain wheatflour.

mechanism is explained more fully later, but essentially diet – specifically FODMAP foods such as wheat, milk and a wide range of fruits and vegetables – will increase this fermentation process, and may contribute to IBS symptoms.

Some FODMAPs may also be 'osmotically active'. This means that when they are left hanging around in the colon, they draw fluid back into it. As one of the colon's main roles is to lose water back into the body to maintain body hydration, FODMAPs that limit this process may result in the looser stools, diarrhoea and urgency associated with IBS.

IBS DIAGNOSIS AND TREATMENT

Because the symptoms of IBS can often be linked to other stomach disorders, it can be quite difficult to diagnose, and it is usually done by process of elimination. Once diagnosed there are then several treatment possibilities.

DIAGNOSIS

There is no one clinical test for IBS – diagnosis is usually made using the internationally agreed 'Rome' criteria, which was set during a conference, held in Rome, by specialist gut doctors (gastroenterologists), medics and dietitians. Before an IBS diagnosis is made using these criteria, the clinician will assess the full clinical picture after other 'red flag' diagnoses have been eliminated. Red flag is a term used to indicate other diseases that may be more worrying, notably cancer. Often simply excluding this will be a huge relief, and sometimes an individual's IBS symptoms may improve just as a result of this removed stress.

THE ROME CRITERIA

These guidelines state that to be diagnosed with IBS, patients should have had symptoms for at least 6 months, and for 3 or more days of the month in the last 3 months. The symptoms should also include abdominal pain or 'discomfort', and be associated with at least 2 of the following:

- Lessening in pain/discomfort when bowels are opened
- A change in bowel frequency since symptoms began
- A change in bowel consistency/form since symptoms began

Other considerations will be any related symptoms, for example stool frequency and type, if there is 'straining' during a bowel movement, or the presence of diarrhoea, mucus or bloating. What is important is that those seeking medical or nutritional advice are appropriately diagnosed and helped. A clear explanation of diagnosis and treatment options by all clinicians is really important so that IBS sufferers have realistic expectations of how they can manage symptoms.

BREATH TESTING

Testing a patient's breath can show how well some sugars – such as fructose or lactose (also FODMAPs) – are actually digested, and can help identify problems with specific foods in IBS. Individuals take a solution of the suspected sugar, and then their exhalation of gases is analysed. Poor digestion of lactose, due to lack of digestive enzyme lactase, means that more lactose will reach the colon. Here 'left over' lactose will be fermented by (healthy) gut bacteria producing gases (hydrogen or methane) that will show up positively on breath tests. While breath testing can be a useful tool to indicate which types of sugars may be contributing to IBS, they aren't always accurate, nor widely available, and are also time consuming.

MEASURING SYMPTOMS

Often in clinical practice IBS symptoms are 'scored' in terms of relative severity on a level between 1 to 10, 10 being the worst, noting how severe each symptom is, or marking this on a visual line scale. This will help you and your dietitian work out what has the biggest impact on your quality of life, and how much your symptoms have improved after a low-FODMAP trial, if at all. You may also be asked about your stool type and frequency, using a visual chart, to help gauge the success of the changes in your diet.

Introduction

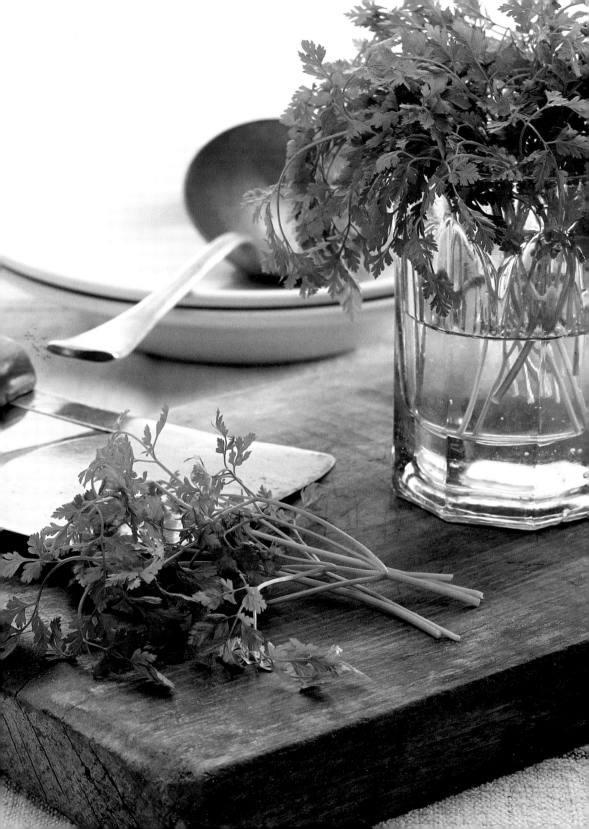

TREATMENT

Since IBS was first recognized it has proved difficult to manage. Doctors have trialled different medications, while dietitians have suggested modifications in diet and lifestyles, and other alternative therapists may also have applied their expertise. The following is an overview of possible treatments.

MEDICATION

The drugs prescribed for IBS are often symptom-based, such as anti-spasmodic (reducing the spasms of gut muscle to reduce pain), anti-diarrhoeal agents, laxatives (if constipated), and even charcoal to help reduce bloating. As with all medicine, there is an element of trial and error, and the review and adjustment of medication can take up much of a doctor's practice time and expense. Bloating in particular – often one of the most distressing aspects of IBS – is rarely improved by medication.

DIET

In the past IBS triggers were not well understood, and diet therapy was focussed on treating symptoms rather than preventing them. Fibre intake may have been encouraged to help those with sluggish bowels, and decreased to help those with urgency and looseness, and today dietary management may still involve this.

Reducing abdominal bloating and wind may have involved limiting the intake of known 'windy' foods including some fruits, vegetables (particularly the brassicas like broccoli and Brussels sprouts), sweeteners, and beans, peas and lentils. Many of us are familiar with the flatulence inevitability of canned baked beans. Food elimination diets have also been used to help establish any intolerances, such as wheat or milk, which may have inadvertently helped. However, none of these treatments were as successful as the low-FODMAP diet has proved to be, which improves symptoms in 70 per cent of patients.

PROBIOTICS AND PREBIOTICS

A probiotic is a natural or commercially produced food that contains healthy gut

Many people feel bloated after eating bread and cakes made with wheat flours.

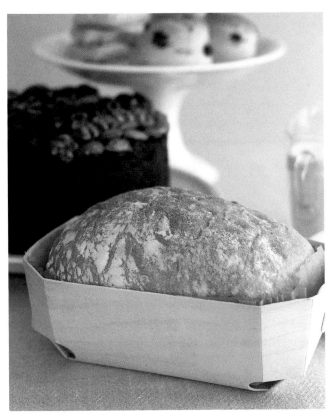

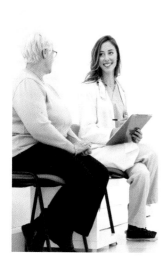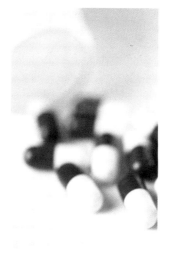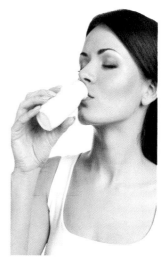

Discussing physical symptoms.   **Probiotics can be taken in capsule form or as a daily drink.**

bacteria aimed to improve health; bacteria may be live, dried or frozen. Prebiotics are natural substances that help 'feed' healthy bacteria in the gut with the aim of creating a similarly healthy environment.

Pro and prebiotics currently hold a prominent and popular place in the health food market and are widely available as commercially produced yogurts or drinks. They can also be bought in tablet or liquid forms, available in pharmacies (drugstores), health food stores, or online.

There still isn't clear scientific evidence for their usefulness in either health or ill health, and many gastroenterologists believe that probiotic bacteria are unable to survive the harsh acidic conditions of the stomach so cannot be of benefit lower down the gut. This does not mean, however, that they have no useful role, and I believe they are worth a personal trial if other interventions have not proved effective. If you decide to test a commercial probiotic, choose one that contains 'good' bacteria such as lactobacilli, or bifidobacter, and take a dosage in line with

product guidance. Also, to help work out any possible benefits of pre or probiotics, it is important not to change any other factors at the same time such as diet or medications, as symptom improvement may be too subtle or otherwise difficult to realize.

ALTERNATIVE THERAPIES

Sufferers understandably wanting quick solutions to their problems may seek alternative treatments including psychotherapy, Cognitive Behavioural Therapy (CBT), hypnotherapy, acupuncture, homeopathy, and more recently 'faecal transplant'. Evidence for the effectiveness of these treatments in IBS is limited, but that does not mean individuals shouldn't consider them if they feel they want to. As with any 'complementary' medicine, do make sure that any practitioner you consult is qualified, and registered with a professional body. Do not be persuaded into potentially damaging treatments such as colonic irrigation, or purchasing expensive supplements or probiotics for which there is no evidence.

LIFESTYLE AND HEALTHY LIVING

Looking after your emotional wellbeing, and eating, sleeping and exercising well could all help manage your IBS. The potential benefits of reducing stress in your life cannot be underestimated, and all of these factors will help to do that.

We have probably all experienced moments when we need to run to the bathroom before an exam or another stressful event, and it may be that the guts of people with IBS are almost permanently (over) stimulated by the routine stresses of daily life that wouldn't affect others. In clinical practice it is always difficult to advise on this, as stress triggers are so individual. Making sufferers aware of this link, however, and helping them acknowledge the affects of busy lives and responsibilities, may prove useful in helping them to manage stress more effectively.

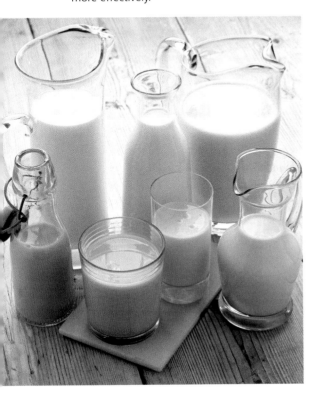

DIGESTIVE ENZYMES

Given that the low-FODMAP diet is about trialling a reduction of poorly digested carbohydrates, it would be logical to wonder whether individuals can't simply take extra digestive enzymes, rather than painstakingly eliminating problem FODMAPs. Scientific trials in this area are very limited, but there is no evidence that they are harmful and I can see potentially useful benefits. As suggested for probiotics, my advice would be to try them if they are affordable. Shop around to find the most effective products, and read reviews to find which brands offer the best value. Enzymes of interest include:

Lactase: this is the enzyme that digests lactose in milk and cheeses. For some years I have seen patients take oral lactase with success, enabling them to digest a limited amount of dairy foods. It is widely available as tablets or drops in health food stores and online. Usually 1–2 tablets (60mg lactase each) are taken per meal. I would certainly recommend a trial of enzyme lactase if it enabled you to consume calcium-rich milk.

Galactosidase: this enzyme digests FODMAPs called galacto-oligosaccharides (GOS), found mainly in beans and pulses. It would therefore be useful for vegetarians wishing to consume these on a low-FODMAP diet that limits intake of beans, pulses and nuts. It costs around the same as lactase, but is less widely available. I would recommend a trial for people who might otherwise miss protein and fibre-rich pulses in their diets.

Xylose isomerase: this enzyme digests fruit sugar, fructose, so potentially could increase an individual's tolerance to fructose-rich fruits and vegetables like apples, stone fruits and asparagus. This is the least widely used of the 3 enzymes suggested, probably due to its expense and limited availability.

Many non-dairy milk substitutes are available.

FODMAPs

While FODMAPs are not the only course of action with IBS management, they are certainly very significant. There is much excitement and anticipation in this area of research, with the success of a low-FODMAP diet becoming globally recognized.

WHAT IS THE LOW-FODMAP DIET?

Interest in FODMAPs started back in 2008 with the publication of an Australian paper showing that there are definite dietary triggers for IBS. In 2010 trials showed that dietary FODMAPs could increase the production of gut gas that can exacerbate IBS symptoms. Excellent-quality research in 2014 confirmed that a low-FODMAP diet does help IBS sufferers, and should be considered as first-line therapy. Gastroenterologists and dietitians from Monash University, Melbourne, and King's College London, continue to work closely together as research develops so that results can be globally shared, and dietitians can help apply this therapy.

To start to understand the diet you will need to have an outline of what the acronym 'FODMAP' stands for. FODMAP is short for 'Fermentable, Oligosaccharides, Disaccharides, Monosaccharides and Polyols', all of which are different types of carbohydrates found in a range of foods. In many people these carbohydrates are easily digested and absorbed, but in IBS sufferers we now understand that they are less well digested, and cause problems in the gut. Their limited digestion is due to a lack of digestive enzymes, which means everyday basic foods like milk or bread have the potential to become FODMAPs. A common example is the lack of the enzyme lactase, causing lactose intolerance that manifests as pain, bloating and looseness when milk is consumed.

The important thing to remember is that a low-FODMAP diet is only a trial, and you'll be discouraged from being on a restrictive diet

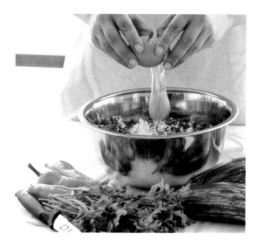

It only takes a few weeks to eliminate FODMAPs.

for any longer than 6–8 weeks. It is possible to have sufficient nutrients on a low-FODMAP diet, but professional help from a dietitian or suitable cookbooks such as this one will be useful. As you'd expect with ongoing research, food lists of restrictive and permissable foods on a low-FODMAP diet will change so it's important to keep up to date. However, at the time of writing there is already a wealth of knowledge proving to be hugely supportive to IBS sufferers worldwide, helping them to achieve a significantly better quality of life.

WHY DO FODMAPs CAUSE PROBLEMS IN IBS?

The process by which bacteria and yeasts feed, by breaking down sugars to make gases and alcohol, is called fermentation; the same key process by which beer and bread are manufactured. The point about FODMAPs is that in IBS sufferers, fermentation is going on in the colon, but it is undesirable. Because they are not fully broken down (digested) in the small intestine (due to lack of suitable enzymes), FODMAPs reach the colon only partially digested, at which point they become a food (fermentation) source for healthy gut bacteria. Fermentation is a natural part of digestion, but in IBS sufferers, too many FODMAPs produce too much gas in the restricted size of the colon. This, combined with the possibility that IBS sufferers have more sensitive guts and feel pain and bloating more than others, is thought to be a significant factor.

Some FODMAPs are also 'osmotically active' so that when they are left 'hanging around' in the colon, they draw fluid back into it, rather than 'losing' it to the body. Osmosis is the process by which water moves from an area of low concentration to high concentration (think how dried fruit swells when soaked in water). As a result there will be too much water in the colon, stools will not be formed, and the diarrhoea and 'urgency' often symptomatic of IBS will result.

WHICH FOODS CONTAIN FODMAPs?

FODMAPs are contained in innocuous, and indeed healthy foods, that we are usually encouraged to eat more of. As you can see in the food table (pages 8–11), FODMAPs include wheat products, dairy foods and a wide range of fruits, vegetables, pulses and nuts. It is therefore not appropriate to think of FODMAP foods as bad or unhealthy, but simply as foods that IBS sufferers absorb less well, and may need to eliminate or eat in smaller quantities.

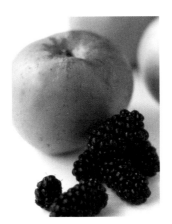

Some fruits are high in FODMAPs.

There are five FODMAP types, which differ only by the length and type of their sugar chains. All have the potential to act as FODMAPs as these structures may not be fully broken down by digestion. Here is an overview of the types of FODMAPs that make up the acronym. Some of these types are further split down (see page 35).

FRUCTANS

These are medium-length chains mainly of fructose molecules, fructose being the sugar commonly found in fruit. From studies it is estimated that most of us do not fully break down these chains during digestion, which means that they end up partially digested in the colon. This is why they can become FODMAPs. Wheat naturally contains fructans, and many foods also contain the fructan 'inulin', which serves as a carbohydrate store in plant foods. Inulin is also used in food manufacturing, as it helps to create a creamy texture without too many calories.

GALACTO-OLIGOSACCHARIDES (GOS)

GOS consist mainly of chains of the sugar galactose, and occur naturally in pulses (beans and lentils), and also in human breastmilk where GOS are a carbohydrate store. Galacto-oligosaccharides are added commercially to foods like infant formula milk, yogurt and breakfast cereals, where they act as a 'prebiotic' encouraging the growth of healthy gut bacteria. In spite of this GOS can also act as a FODMAP and create potential IBS symptoms though excess gas production and trapped wind.

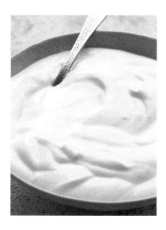

Although milk is quite limited, cream can be included.

DISACCHARIDES

Sugars consisting of just two molecules are called disaccharides and include lactose, commonly known as 'milk sugar'. Lactose needs the gut enzyme 'lactase' in order to be digested, but often this is in low supply or lacking due to hereditary factors, or diseases that may have damaged the gut such as Coeliac or Crohn's disease. Studies have shown that some people with IBS have less lactase, which means that milk (lactose) could become a FODMAP as its digestion will be limited. Lactose is also used in drugs, and in food manufacturing as a 'filler', or to improve the colour of baked goods.

MONOSACCHARIDES

Sugars consisting of just one molecule are called monosaccharides and include fructose, the predominant sugar in fruit. Fructose is used in food manufacturing as it is naturally sweeter than white sugar (sucrose). It also has a lower glycaemic index (meaning it raises blood sugar levels more slowly on digestion), so is favoured by the slimming industry. Fructose is a common FODMAP.

Interestingly though, unlike other FODMAPs, the potential for fructose to cause IBS gut symptoms is considerably affected by the amount of glucose (a monosaccharide) contained within the same food. This is because glucose helps 'carry' the fructose molecule across the gut wall, so it is the glucose/fructose ratio that determines how much of a problem fructose-containing foods will be.

POLYOLS

Also known as 'sugar alcohols' polyols are where oxygen and hydrogen molecules are attached to a sugar molecule. A well-known polyol is 'sorbitol', a sweetener used in diabetic foods, gum and laxatives. Mannitol is another less well-known sugar alcohol found in watermelon, cauliflower and sweet potato.

Stone fruits must be avoided, but most natural sugar is permitted.

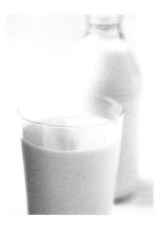

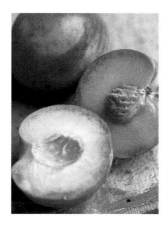

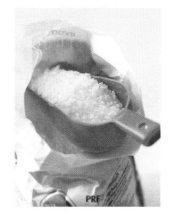

STARTING A LOW-FODMAP DIET

A low-FODMAP trial takes part in two phases, an initial elimination phase over four to eight weeks, followed by a re-introduction phase over a similar time, where suspect foods are reintroduced into the diet to assess tolerance.

ELIMINATION PHASE

During the four to eight weeks of elimination, FODMAP-rich foods are removed completely from the diet (any food in the red column of the food table on pages 8–11), or eaten in moderation (food in the yellow column) if possible. Foods in the green column contain negligible or no FODMAPs, and can be eaten freely. Following the diet takes some thought, planning and vigilance, and while I have enjoyed some successes with patients I have also found some who have decided the diet is too difficult. Making sure that you understand the theory, choosing a suitable time to start, and preparing adequately will all help. Avoid following the diet at a time when you have social commitments or holidays, as eating out on a low-FODMAP diet can be challenging. Ideally you would follow the diet strictly for the full trial period, as breaking it, even for one meal, makes it difficult to assess its effect.

Access to a FODMAP-trained dietitian is also helpful as he/she will be well versed in any changes to food lists (which are continually evolving), and can tailor advice to your individual medical and personal needs. A dietitian will also help you 'score' your symptoms. Comparing these with scores at the end of your trial will help gauge any improvements from the diet.

In the majority there are clear improvements after the trial: less pain, firmer stools, and loss of urgency, and the results can be quite life-changing. If a low-FODMAP diet is right for you, you should see some improvement after 2–4 weeks, if you are not sure of the results then I would suggest continuing for a further 2–4 weeks. If there is still no improvement, it is likely that the diet isn't going to help your IBS, and you might have to seek alternative strategies ideally with the support of a doctor. Hopefully, however, you will see a change, and can go on to a re-introduction phase.

RESOURCES

Professionally prepared diet sheets are available though may only be distributed through dietitians to help protect accuracy

TIPS FOR SUCCESS

Keeping these tips in mind while you are in the elimination stage will increase your success rates.
• Preparation is key. Take a few days to make sure you have suitable foods at home, which will help you stick to the diet. Stock up on everyday staple alternatives before you begin.
• Remember that many everyday foods are suitable; fresh meat, fish, eggs, oils and butters, hard cheeses, potatoes, rice, and a good range of vegetables and salads are all FODMAP-free, and are great for putting together quick meals.
• Caffeine is fine in moderation (2–3 cups daily), and you can include up to 50ml/2fl oz/¼ cup milk per day in tea or coffee.
• You can include a limited amount of wine, beer and spirits in your elimination phase, but not rum or dessert wines.

Introduction

HIGH-FODMAP FOODS, AND SUITABLE LOW-FODMAP ALTERNATIVES

Preparing your store cupboard for a low-FODMAP trial will help you complete it without too much difficulty. This table shows handy alternatives to everyday foods that you'd have to exclude on the trial.

HIGH-FODMAP FOOD	LOW-FODMAP ALTERNATIVE
Cow, sheep and goat's milks	Soya, nut, rice, coconut and lactose-free milks. Most people with lactose intolerance can manage up to 50ml/2fl oz/¼ cup regular cow's (or other mammalian) milk in hot drinks through the day
Regular wheat-based bread, cakes, biscuits, cookies	Wheat-free commercial alternatives, corn tortillas, oatcakes, home baking made with suitable flours
Regular wheat pasta	Wheat-free pasta, block polenta, rice, quinoa, buckwheat, potato
Regular wheat-based cereals, eg muesli (granola), branflakes, wheat biscuits	Oat or corn-based cereals such as wheat-free muesli, rolled oats, cornflakes, puffed rice
Onions, garlic, leeks, spring onions (scallions), white parts	Spring onion, green part only, garlic-infused oil (no garlic pieces), asafoetida powder, regular herbs and spices
Wheat flour in sauces	Cornflour (cornstarch)
Regular stock (bouillon) cubes/gravy powder containing onion and garlic	Onion/garlic free stock cubes (if available) or homemade stock
Fruit such as apple, pear, watermelon	Clementines, grapes, galia melon, banana, strawberries, raspberries
Fruit juice/sports drinks containing sorbitol/fructose	Limit fruit juice to 100ml/3½fl oz/scant ½ cup (suitable fruits only). Add carbonated water, 30ml/2 tbsp maple syrup and 2.5ml/½ tsp salt for a homemade sports drink
Dessert wine/rum	Regular red or white wine, spirits other than rum, beer or ale

Introduction

and quality. Monash University also has an excellent FODMAP app that suggests suitable foods using a 'traffic light' system, and provides recipes with 'filters' for FODMAP types. Be wary of online FODMAP advice unless it has an academic origin as many have created websites with untested food lists, and providing advice of dubious accuracy.

VEGETARIANS AND VEGANS

Omitting beans, pulses, and some vegetables and nuts on a low-FODMAP trial can reduce a vegetarian or vegan's intake of essential amino acids (proteins). With careful planning, however, these can be replaced by eating suitable vegetables, nuts, eggs, soya mince (TVP), wheat-free Quorn (TM), and nutritious pulses such as quinoa, buckwheat and wholegrain rice. Professional, tailored advice would be useful, particularly for vegans.

BAKING

There are a wide range of wheat-free flours that can be successfully used in baking, and often specially blended commercial blends will produce the best results. Xanthan gum, made

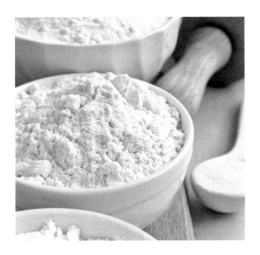

from the fermentation of 'good' bacteria, improves the elasticity, flavour and stability of wheat-free flours that are low in gluten, and is FODMAP-friendly. Guar gum, made from the seeds of an Indian legume plant, has similar properties. Other useful wheat-free ingredients for baking are ground nuts (taking into account restrictions on portion sizes), polenta (cornmeal) and cornflour (cornstarch). Gram (chickpea), soya, millet or pea flours, though all are wheat-free, must be avoided in a low-FODMAP trial.

Not all gluten-free flours are suitable for the diet.

SUITABLE LOW-FODMAP FLOURS

On a low-FODMAP diet, you will need to exclude regular wheat flour and related products. The range of wheat-free alternatives is increasing, and you can of course buy suitable flours and have creative fun in the kitchen. This table shows alternative suitable flours for using in a low-FODMAP diet, and gives ideas for using them.

TYPE	PROPERTIES
Arrowroot	A fine flour derived from the plantain family, useful for making thick, clear glazes.
Buckwheat	A wholegrain flour with an attractive calico colour, and natural sweetness, which is pleasant in pancakes, noodles and baking.
Chestnut flour	A flour with natural sweetness useful for baking. It has a low carbohydrate content, but useful levels of protein.
Cornflour (cornstarch)	Cornflour is an excellent substitute for wheat flour to thicken sauces and gravy, and can also be used to coat foods before light frying, or in baking.
Oat flour	Oat flour can be easily made by grinding regular oats in a food processor. It is a satisfying coarse-textured flour useful for pancakes and baking.
Potato flour	Also known as potato 'farina', this starchy flour can be mixed with cold water and used to thicken soups, batters or breads.
Quinoa flour	Buttery, yellow, quinoa flour is protein- and fat-rich. It makes excellent baked goods, though pastry needs delicate handling.
Rice flour	A versatile staple in many Asian cuisines for making noodles and desserts, rice flour is also useful as a thickener in sauces and gravies, and for lighter baking results.
Sago flour	A starchy flour, derived from the sago palm in Southeast Asia, that can be used for thickening and baking.
Tapioca flour	This is made from grinding the dried roots of the cassava plant, and can be used in breads and for thickening sauces.
Flour blends	Commercial flour blends made from a range of the above and often pre-mixed with Xanthan gum, are widely available and designed for successful wheat-free baking

MAINTAINING A LOW-FODMAP DIET

A low-FODMAP trial should last between four to eight weeks. Since this isn't an insignificant amount of time, here is some practical advice on how to achieve this, with some help on adapting recipes that you can still enjoy.

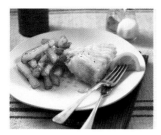 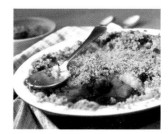 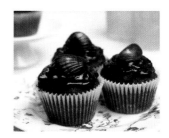

ADAPTING FAVOURITE RECIPES

The table below gives you examples of how to adapt recipes. Of course this does take a bit more time and thought, but using the principles below, together with the food tables, and making sure that you have storecupboard essentials, will help. You will also find lots of inspiration and new ideas from the recipe chapters to help you stick it out!

FODMAP-RICH RECIPES	LOW FODMAP ALTERNATIVE
Macaroni cheese	Use wheat-free pasta. Make a cheese sauce using recipe on page 39. Avoid lactose-rich soft cheeses.
Pepperoni pizza	Make pizza dough using wheat-free flour. Cover with onion-free passata (bottled strained tomatoes), mozzarella and ham or chicken and herbs. Spice up with chilli oil.
Roast chicken dinner	Chicken, potatoes, carrots and parsnips are fine. Make onion-free gravy with meat juices. Eat allowed amounts of peas, broccoli and corn.
Fish pie	Place the fish in an ovenproof dish and cover with a mixture of mascarpone and crème fraîche, cover with cheesy mashed potato and bake.
Meatloaf	Use your usual recipe but flavour the meat with herbs and spring onion greens instead of garlic and onion. Bind with egg and cornflour (cornstarch) instead of flour and include FODMAP-friendly vegetables.
Vegetable lasagne	Use wheat-free lasagne. Make cheese sauce as per recipe on page 39. Use soya mince (TVP), passata and suitable vegetables. Top with mozzarella.
Apple crumble and custard	Use rhubarb, or raspberry and banana. Make crumble using wheat-free flour and oats. Make custard using milk alternative.
Fruit fool	Poach your favourite low-FODMAP fruit in a little liquid, then fold through lightly whipped double (heavy) cream. Chill thoroughly and then serve in tall glasses topped with flaked (sliced) almonds.
Chocolate muffins	Make muffins using wheat-free flour and cocoa powder. Replace buttermilk with cream. Use plain (semisweet) chocolate chips.

EATING OUT

This is definitely more tricky on a low-FODMAP trial as, inevitably, restaurant and hotel dishes will be packed full of onion, garlic and wheat-based pastry, pasta and breads. However 'allergen' labelling is definitely improving with many countries now requiring this at the point of sale, including restaurants. Unfortunately following the trial does take some spontaneity out of eating out, but if you can plan and pre-order I think you will be pleasantly surprised with the possibilities. Many pizza and pasta restaurants now serve wheat-free as a matter of course, and teamed up with suitable cheeses, meat, fish and vegetables you can enjoy a tasty supper, even with a glass of wine and salad on the side. If you can access the 'Monash' FODMAP App on your smartphone, you'll find it easy to check foods, but if not keep your list of unsuitable ingredients handy for checking.

- Choose meat and fish flavoured with herbs and seasonings, and a side of potatoes/rice and vegetables or salad
- Avoid soups, sauces, gravies, stuffing, pastry, dumplings and breaded foods
- Vegetarian dishes must be carefully checked for hidden pulses and unsuitable nuts

- Stick to risottos, omelettes and casseroles made with suitable vegetables, and top generously with tasty mature (sharp) cheeses
- Indian, Chinese and Mexican foods tend to contain a lot of onion and garlic, you're probably better avoiding or making at home
- Platters of meat, fish, sun-dried peppers, olives and most salad items can been eaten freely, but you'll need to avoid bread
- For desserts choose berries, pineapple, meringues with cream, or ice cream

SNACKS AND LUNCHBOXES

You will probably find that you will become more reliant on taking your own food for the period of the trial. Having the confidence to know that you can eat quickly in your work break, without relying on food outlets, will be a bonus even if it means advance preparation. Here are some lunchbox ideas, some of which may be leftovers from dinner the day before.

FRUIT AND NUTS
- Sliced banana with Greek (strained plain) yogurt
- Small handful dried fruit and suitable nuts (except pistachio nuts/cashew nuts)
- Fresh berries, citrus, pineapple

With a little preparation and forward planning it is quite easy to take a low-FODMAP lunch to work.

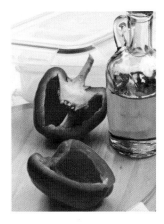
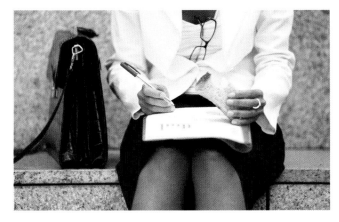

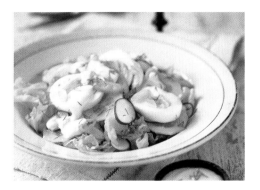

Lettuce and egg salad.

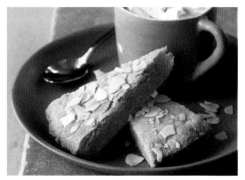

Polenta cake.

VEGETABLES AND DIPS
- Homemade carrot and coriander soup
- Aubergine (eggplant) dip served with oatcakes
- Carrot, courgette (zucchini) and (bell) pepper crudités with a sour cream and herb dip
- ½ small roasted sweet potato with blue cheese and wilted spinach

'CARBS' AND TOPPINGS
- Rice cakes with brie and yeast extract
- Oatcakes with peanut butter
- Corn tortilla tacos or chips filled with grated cheese, salad and sour cream
- Wheat-free bread filled with chicken or egg mayonnaise and cucumber
- Rice noodles tossed with canned salmon, fish sauce and wilted spinach

PORTABLE MEALS
- Cold, sliced radicchio frittata
- Roast (bell) peppers, halloumi and pine nuts
- Lettuce and egg salad
- Pasta salad made from wheat-free pasta, cooked chicken, broccoli, passata (bottled strained tomatoes) and grated cheese
- Rice salad made with tuna, corn and soy sauce (hot or cold)
- Hard-boiled egg
- Take-out sushi (check ingredients)
- Beef sandwich made from gluten-free bread

SWEET TREATS
- Polenta cake
- Dark (bittersweet) chocolate
- Up to 30g/1¼oz white/milk chocolate
- Wheat-free cookies/cakes

DRINKS
- Suitable carbonated water, drinks or cordial, check for sweeteners ending in '- ol', and 'unsuitable' fruits eg peach or apple. Lemon and lime are good
- Tea/coffee/chocolate with a dash of regular milk or milk substitute for a milkier drink

FREQUENTLY ASKED QUESTIONS

Here are some common questions often asked by IBS sufferers about the low-FODMAP diet.

Will I get enough nutrients on a low-FODMAP trial?

Because the diet is low in wheat products, and limits some fruit and vegetables and milk, it is possible your fibre and calcium intake will decrease. Take a daily multivitamin with calcium (approximately 400mg), eat five portions of low-FODMAP fruit and vegetables a day, and boost your calcium intake with canned fish, oranges, sesame seeds and spinach. Don't try the diet if you are pregnant, trying to conceive, or breast feeding.

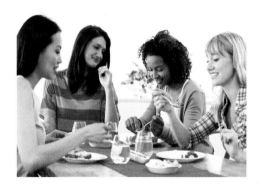

Can I follow the diet if I'm a vegetarian/vegan

Most vegetarian protein sources, such as eggs, tofu, tempeh, soya mince, some cheeses and most nuts (see food lists) are fine on a low-FODMAP diet. Just avoid cooking them with unsuitable vegetables. Vegans may find the diet more challenging as all pulses and lentils, cashews and pistachios need excluding. However, you should be able to get adequate protein from suitable vegetables, grains such as rice and quinoa, tofu, tempeh, quorn, soya mince, seeds and most nuts.

Is the diet suitable for diabetics?

A low-FODMAP diet should contain adequate starchy carbohydrates in the form of rice, potato, wheat-free bread and suitable grains, so hypoglycaemia should not be a risk. Because polyols such as sorbitol and xylitol should be excluded from a low-FODMAP trial, however, it is important that diabetics who regularly include these in diet drinks and confectionery do not switch to high sugar alternatives. Although regular sugar (sucrose) is not a FODMAP, intake should clearly not be encouraged on a low-FODMAP trial in those with diabetes. Similarly, your intake of suitable fruits should be limited to 2–3 portions a day to limit any excess rise in blood sugar levels. Eat plenty of low-FODMAP vegetables or salads instead.

Eat in with friends rather than in restaurants.

Will a low-FODMAP affect my weight?

Cutting down on major food groups like wheat and dairy may result in weight loss if the diet isn't suitably balanced elsewhere. However, if you are trying to lose weight, it is best not to focus on calorie control during the low-FODMAP trial as your diet may become too low in vital vitamins and minerals. If you are overweight, limit your intake of fatty foods. Commit to regular activity such as walking and gardening, or more vigorous running, gym or swimming if you are able. If you are underweight, or have a tendency to lose weight easily, include plenty of FODMAP-friendly meat, fish, potatoes, rice and grains, nuts and suitable cheeses to help limit this.

Can I still exercise?

There is no reason why a low-FODMAP trial should adversely affect your energy levels, or ability to exercise, so long as it remains balanced. Eat plenty of slow-release carbs to help build up muscle glycogen stores, such as porridge, wholegrain basmati rice, grains such as buckwheat and quinoa, and wheat-free pasta. Before exercise eat some quick-release sugars in the form of suitable fruit (banana, clementines or grapes), a handful of raisins or rice cakes. Don't use sports drinks that often contain sugar alcohols such as sorbitol or xylitol, which are FODMAPs.

Is the diet suitable for children?

IBS in children is not currently well recognized, though other food allergy and elimination diets, other than FODMAPs, are used in clinical practice. No child should be put on to an elimination diet without specialist dietetic input, as weight and other markers would need to be closely monitored. That said, feeding your family a few low-FODMAP meals during your trial should be fine.

RE-INTRODUCTION OF FODMAPs

After the low-FODMAP trial you should begin to introduce potentially offending foods back into your diet (the re-introduction phase) in a controlled way. This will help you work out which FODMAPs you are sensitive to.

The ultimate aim of this process is to maximize the range of foods and nutrients you can eat while managing IBS symptoms. Some individuals feel so well after completing their low-FODMAP trial, that they are understandably reluctant to start the re-introduction phase, which may worsen their symptoms. However re-introduction should be encouraged because a long-term low-FODMAP diet is likely to be nutritionally restricted, often lacking in calcium and fibre. Permanent low-FODMAP eating also poses practical challenges in everyday social eating and cooking.

Re-introduction often shows that it is only 1 or 2 types of foods that cause problems, and hopefully in the long term this gives you the scope to start relaxing more with the diet, enjoying a wider range of foods. You may also learn that you have different tolerances for FODMAP foods, for example you can manage milk and bread in small amounts, but they cause problems in larger quantities. Cumulative intake of the same types of FODMAPs may also cause problems, for example a breakfast consisting of milk in tea and a serving of yogurt, which may cause bloating as a result of too much lactose, but eaten separately would be fine. Likewise with fructose, where too many limited fruits – for example grapes and clementines at the same time – might cause problems in a fruit salad, but individually would be fine.

TYPES OF FODMAPs IN FOODS
To help with the re-introduction phase, and assess your own individual tolerances, you need to have an idea of what FODMAPs

individual foods contain. The table on page 35 doesn't include all foods listed in the table on pages 8–11, as FODMAP breakdowns are not always available, but gives enough of a range to work out what FODMAPs cause problems.

STARTING RE-INTRODUCTION
The re-introduction phase can be slightly more relaxed than the elimination diet, but it is still advisable to limit potential interruptions as

Rice is a great stand-by food for both phases.

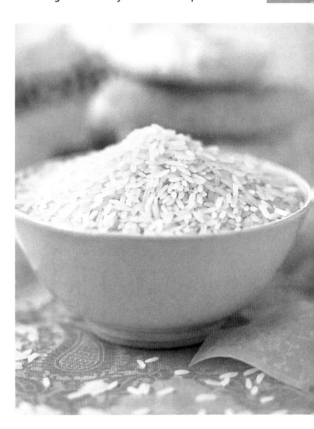

much as possible. The idea is that you will still be eating a 'baseline' low-FODMAP diet through the elimination phase, so eating out and holidays will still need consideration. If you are trying to assess the effect of including FODMAP-rich foods, it is helpful to try and limit other factors that may also affect the way your gut functions, so lower your intake of caffeine, alcohol and spicy foods, and keep your stress levels low. If your symptoms worsen after reintroducing a particular food you need to allow a 'washout' period of a day between the next test, to allow your gut to settle down and flush out any problem foods.

You can test GOS, fructose, lactose and polyols in one go, that is you only need to try one type of food from that group to see if you can manage other FODMAPs in the same group. For example you will see from the table opposite that you can select broccoli or avocado to challenge polyol (sorbitol). The exception to this is fructans, which each need to be challenged separately, as each individual's gut handles them differently. You will therefore need to test each individual type

of fructans that you wish to re-include, for example bread, flour, wheat-based cereals, peaches etc.

Some foods such as mushrooms contain two or more types of FODMAPs – fructans and polyols – but there is no need to test these more than once.

There is less scientific evidence about the exact detail of re-introducing foods, but the following guidelines work well in my everyday practice so I can recommend them. Use the table below to guide you in testing which FODMAP foods may cause you problems. After the staged re-introduction you may find that you can tolerate certain FODMAPs at lower levels. This seems often to be the case with onion and garlic (fructans), which can cause wind, bloating and pain in large quantities. What is important is that you feel empowered to manage IBS through diet without making difficult dietary restrictions.

Garlic, and onions of any type, are to be avoided completely during the elimination phase.

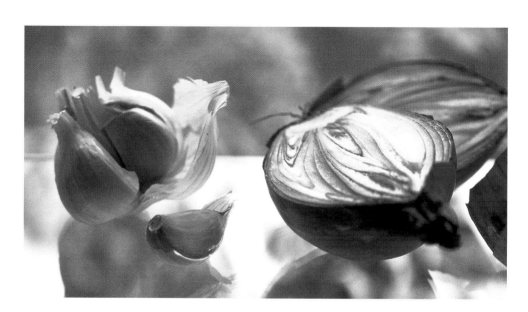

FODMAP TYPES

FRUCTANS

Almonds	Chicory	Leeks	Prunes
Amaranth	Chicory root	Mangetouts (snow peas)	Raisins
Apricots	Coconut water	Mushrooms	Rye
Artichokes	Cranberries	Nectarines	Savoy cabbage
Asparagus	Dandelion tea	Okra	Spelt
Barley	Dates	Onions	Spring onions (scallions)
Beetroot (beets)	Fennel	Oolong tea	(white part)
Brussels sprouts	Fennel tea	Peaches	Stone fruits: all, also as
Cashew nuts	Figs (dried)	Pistachio nuts	desserts, cordials etc
Chai	Garlic	Plums	Watermelons
Chamomile tea	Grapefruit	Pomegranates	Wheat

GOS (Galacto Oligosaccharides)

Almonds	Butternut squash	Mangetouts (snow peas)	Rye
Amaranth	Carob Powder	Peas	Wheat
Barley	Cashew nuts	Persimmon	
Beans and pulses (all)	Corn	Pistachio nuts	

LACTOSE (Disaccharides)

Buttermilk	Evaporated, condensed	Low-fat cheeses	Soft cheeses
Cottage cheese	milk	Milk (any animal,	Yogurts
Cream cheese	Fromage frais	all fat types)	
Custard	Ice cream	Processed cheese slices	

FRUCTOSE (Monosaccharides)

Apples	Cashew nuts	Honey	Pistachio nuts
Artichoke hearts	Cherries	Jerusalem artichokes	Rum
Asparagus	Dessert wines	Mangoes	Rye
Bananas (very ripe)	Figs	Pears (dried)	Sugar snap peas
Boysenberries	Grapefruit	Pineapples (dried)	Watermelons

POLYOL (Sorbitol)

Apples	Broccoli	Corn	Pears
Apricots	Cherries	Lychees	Plums
Avocados	Coconuts	Nectarines	Prunes
Blackberries	Coconut water	Peaches	Sugar-free gum

POLYOL (Mannitol)

Butternut squash	Fennel bulb	Sugar-free gum
Cauliflower	Mangetouts (snow peas)	Sweet potatoes
Celery	Mushrooms	Watermelons

GUIDELINES FOR RE-TESTING INDIVIDUAL FODMAPs

- Before you start re-introduction, decide which foods you need to test so that you can work out how long this will take you. Each food needs a test period of 3 days, so if you're testing 10 foods you need 30 days, plus a potential 2 3-day washouts, giving a total of 36 days. This will help you plan to avoid holidays or social events, should you get a 'reaction' to a food.
- Test foods over a 3-day period, doubling the amount each day, to help you gauge your individual tolerances.
- Remember that you don't have to eat all of the test food at the same time. Spread intake of the test foods throughout the day if this is more practical and tolerable.
- Even if you find foods that are acceptable during the re-introduction phase, it is recommended that your diet remains FODMAP-free as much as possible until you've tested all the foods, as there might be incremental effects of FODMAPs, ie onion with other fructans.
- If you find a food that worsens your IBS, stop eating it and begin the 3-day washout period before testing another food. This means you should go back to a baseline low-FODMAP diet.
- During the re-introduction keep a simple food and symptom diary detailing foods challenged, and symptoms experienced. We have included a template on page 45 for you to photocopy or scan and fill in. Symptoms indicate that FODMAPs in your test food have caused you problems, and it is unlikely that you will be able to tolerate that food in your diet. However, you can always re-test this in the future.
- Use scores of individual symptoms to help you remember which foods you have problems with, and what your personal tolerance levels are.
- Lastly, remember that re-introduction isn't an exact science. Use your common sense, or consult a dietitian if you are unsure about symptoms or foods.

TEST FOODS FOR RE-INTRODUCTION

FODMAP TO TEST	TEST FOODS TO USE	AMOUNTS RECOMMENDED
Fructans	Test individual foods such as apple, wheat, pasta, pistachios	Day 1: eat a third of the amount that you'd normally, then double and triple this by day 3
GOS (Oligosaccharides)	Any beans or pulses such as lentils, chickpeas, broad (fava) beans, peas	Day 1: 45ml/2 tbsp, increasing to 90ml/6 tbsp by day 3
Lactose (Disaccharides)	Regular milk or yogurt without FODMAP fruit	Day 1: 120ml/4fl oz/½ cup milk or 125g/4¼oz yogurt, increasing to 375g/13oz by day 3
Fructose (Mono-saccharides)	Mango, honey	Day 1: ½ mango or 5ml/1 tsp honey, increasing to 1½ mangoes, 15ml/1 tbsp honey by day 3
Polyol (Sorbitol)	Broccoli or avocado	Day 1: 3 x small florets broccoli or ¼ avocado, increasing to 9 small florets or a whole small avocado by day 3
Polyol (Mannitol)	Cauliflower, celery or sweet potato	Day 1: 2 small florets of cauliflower or 1 celery stick or 45ml/3 tbsp cooked sweet potato, increasing to 6 florets of cauliflower, 3 celery sticks or 1 small sweet potato by day 3

LOW-FODMAP ALTERNATIVE BASIC RECIPES

Finding suitable condiments and sauces is tricky on a low-FODMAP diet, as many contain onion and garlic. With improved labelling, it is easier to find FODMAP-free products but these homemade versions will help keep your diet varied.

HARISSA PASTE

Onions and garlic are usually included in this North African spice mixture, but this alternative is just as fiery and vibrant. Use to flavour soups and stews.

Brush the peppers and chillies with 15ml/1 tbsp of the oil, and grill (broil), skin-side up, until softened. Turn the grill (broiler) to high for a further few minutes to blacken slightly.

Meanwhile heat the rest of the oil in a small pan, and add the remaining ingredients except the lemon juice and yogurt. Lightly fry for 2–3 minutes, using the end of a rolling pin to crush the seeds and release the flavours.

Add the spice mix to a food processor with the chillies and peppers, lemon juice, yogurt and a good pinch of salt. Blitz until semi-coarse, or smoother if preferred. Transfer to a clean jar, seal and keep in the refrigerator. Use within 1 week.

COOK'S TIP If you haven't got a food processor, use a pestle and mortar to blend the ingredients together.

2 red (bell) peppers, halved and deseeded
2 red chillies, halved and deseeded
30ml/2 tbsp olive or other vegetable oil
2.5ml/½ tsp asafoetida powder
2.5ml/½ tsp cumin seeds
2.5ml/½ tsp coriander seeds
2.5ml/½ tsp paprika
2.5ml/½ tsp dried chilli flakes
30ml/2 tbsp lemon juice
45ml/3 tbsp natural (plain) yogurt
salt

THAI YELLOW CURRY PASTE

Lemon grass stalk and shrimp paste blend with spices to make this fragrant paste. Use with coconut milk or stock to make a rich curry, or use to coat meat or fish.

10ml/2 tsp hot chilli powder
10ml/2 tsp ground coriander
10ml/2 tsp ground cumin
5ml/1 tsp turmeric
30ml/2 tbsp finely chopped lemon grass stalk
5ml/1 tsp shrimp paste (optional)
5ml/1 tsp finely grated lime rind
60ml/4 tbsp vegetable oil

Combine all of the ingredients. Store in an airtight container in the refrigerator and use within 2–3 weeks.

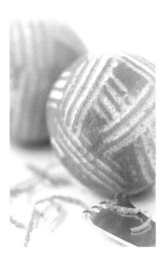

THAI SWEET CHILLI SAUCE

120ml/4fl oz/½ cup rice or
    white wine vinegar
100g/3¾oz/½ cup sugar
60ml/4 tbsp water
45ml/3 tbsp fish sauce
30ml/2 tbsp sherry
15ml/1 tbsp dried chilli flakes
15ml/1 tbsp cornflour
    (cornstarch), mixed with
    15ml/1 tbsp cold water

This dipping sauce can be a great staple in your low-FODMAP store cupboard, ideal for those that like a 'kick' to their food. This recipe makes 3–4 servings, and it will keep in the refrigerator for 2–3 weeks, so double up for a larger quantity.

Place all the ingredients, apart from the cornflour mixture, into a medium pan. Simmer for 8–10 minutes over a low heat until reduced by approximately a half.

Remove from the heat, and add 30ml/2 tbsp of the liquid from the pan to the cornflour mixture to blend. Then return the pan to the heat and, stirring quickly, add the cornflour mixture to the pan, cook for 1–2 minutes, stirring, to thicken. The sauce should be the consistency of a thin syrup. Cool and use as a dip. Keep in a sealed container in the refrigerator.

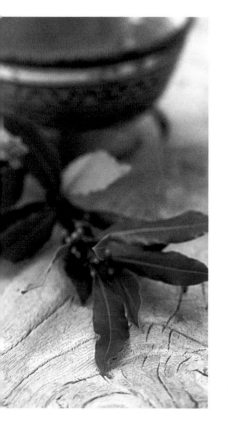

VEGETABLE STOCK

Finding onion and garlic-free stock (bouillon) cubes is possible, though challenging, and it is much easier to make your own. This simple recipe for vegetable stock can be used in curries, soups and casseroles. Do substitute other FODMAP-friendly vegetables and fresh herbs, depending on what you have to hand.

pinch asafoetida powder
15ml/1 tbsp garlic-infused oil
1 celery stick, or bunch spring
    onions (scallions), green part
    only, cut into slices
1 carrot, peeled and sliced
750ml/1½ pints/3 cups boiling
    water

5ml/1 tsp yeast extract or
    soy sauce
3 bay leaves
small bunch parsley, including
    stalks
2.5ml/½ tsp salt
black pepper, to taste

Heat the asafoetida with the oil for 2–3 minutes on a low heat, then add the vegetables and fry for a further couple of minutes to soften.

Add the remaining ingredients and simmer for 15–20 minutes, stirring occasionally until the vegetables are tender. Strain the reserved stock, discarding the vegetables. Keep in the refrigerator or freeze, and use as required.

CHICKEN STOCK

Make great use of a roasted chicken carcass, or an uncooked one from your butcher, to make this delicious low-FODMAP chicken stock. Freeze in ice-cube trays, if you wish, for stock cube substitutes, or use in one go for a soup or risotto.

30ml/2 tbsp garlic-infused oil
2.5ml/½ tsp asafoetida powder
3 peeled carrots, diced
4 spring onions (scallions), green part only, roughly chopped
1 whole chicken carcass, raw or roasted

2 bay leaves
10ml/2 tsps dried mixed herbs, or a handful fresh chopped herbs such as thyme or oregano
5ml/1 tsp salt
black pepper

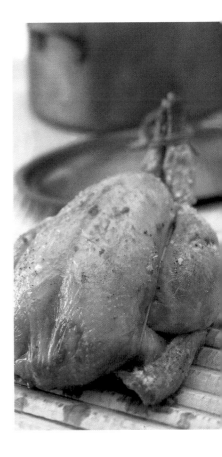

In a large casserole dish, heat the oil with the asafoetida powder for 2–3 minutes to release the flavour. Add the carrots and spring onion greens, and soften for 2 minutes, then add the chicken carcass and add enough water to just cover.

Bring to the boil, add the remaining ingredients, and simmer for approximately 45 minutes to 1 hour, stirring occasionally. Strain the stock, discard the vegetables and leave to cool. Use as desired, or freeze. The stock will keep covered in the refrigerator for 2–3 days.

CHEESE SAUCE

Based on a classic béchamel, this cheese sauce uses cornflour for thickening and is beautifully rich and creamy. Use it to make macaroni cheese or for use on any wheat-free pasta, low-FODMAP vegetables or fish.

45g/1½oz/¼ cup cornflour (cornstarch)
550ml/18fl oz/2½ cups low-FODMAP vegetable stock
60ml/4 tbsp double (heavy) cream
115g/4oz mature (sharp) Cheddar cheese, grated
pinch mustard powder
salt and black pepper

Blend the cornflour with 60ml/4 tbsp of the cold stock, then warm the rest of the stock in a pan.

Add the cornflour mixture to the pan, whisking to blend, then bring to the boil, stirring on a medium heat until thickened, then add the cream.

Remove the pan from the heat, and add the grated Cheddar cheese, mustard and seasoning to taste. Stir until the cheese is melted, returning to the heat if necessary. The sauce is now ready to use.

ELIMINATION WEEKLY EATING PLANS

The following eating plans offer ideas for meals and snacks to eat while following a low-FODMAP trial; they can be mixed and matched as desired and are suggestions rather than strict guidelines. If time is short in the mornings, stick to breakfast staples such as porridge or wheat-free toast, but we've also included recipes for more creative moments. Drinks should remain as simple as possible such as water, tea and coffee, and suitable cordials such as lemon or lime. Please refer to the FODMAPs list at the front of this chapter, on pages 8–11, to make sure that you don't go over the recommended amounts of limited foods where included.

TWO-WEEK LOW-FODMAP PLAN

	BREAKFAST/BRUNCH	LUNCH	SUPPER	SNACKS
SATURDAY	Bacon and Cheese Cornbread Muffins (page 57)	Chicken and Lemon Soup (page 66)	Baked Bream (page 87) with green beans and carrots, Baked Bananas with Toffee Sauce (page 155)	Wheat-free biscuit (cookie)
SUNDAY	Salmon and Quinoa Frittata (page 55)	Paprika Pork (page 121) with spicy potato wedges and 3 asparagus spears	Polenta Cake (page 170) with crème fraîche	
MONDAY	Granola (page 49) served with 30ml/ 2 tbsp Greek (strained plain) yogurt	Oatcakes with peanut butter or Cheddar cheese and cucumber	Beef Pie with Potato Crust (page 115), small portion broccoli and roast parsnips	Courgette and Ginger Cake (page 172)
TUESDAY	Wheat-free toast with peanut butter or butter and yeast extract	Carrot and Coriander Soup (page 71)	Tuscan-style Chicken (page 111) with Polenta Chips (page 79) and a small portion peas, Blueberry Parfait (page 162)	Slice of galia melon
WEDNESDAY	Porridge made with low-lactose milk	Salt and Pepper Fried Squid (page 80), 1 tomato and cucumber	Radicchio Frittata (page 133) with new potatoes	Raspberry Friands (page 169)
THURSDAY	30ml/2 tbsp natural (plain) yogurt with a sliced banana and a Blueberry Muffin (page 60)	Tuna with Polenta (page 88)	Miso Soup with Pork (page 73)	Few squares plain (semi sweet) chocolate
FRIDAY	Cornflakes/puffed rice with low-lactose milk and sliced strawberries	Rice, Buckwheat and Corn Bread (page 173) with Camembert and a few grapes	Spaghetti with Tuna, Anchovies and Capers (page 92)	30ml/2 tbsp natural yogurt with sliced banana

Introduction

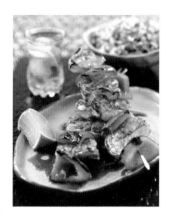
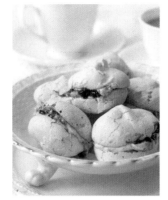
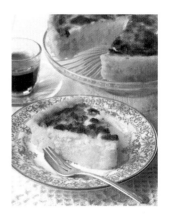

	BREAKFAST/BRUNCH	LUNCH	SUPPER	SNACKS
SATURDAY	Buckwheat Pancakes with Grilled Bacon (page 56)	Ham salad served with wheat-free pitta	Tapenade with Quail Eggs and Crudités (page 74) Tangy Prawn Kebabs (page 101) with rice	Sliced orange
SUNDAY	Oat Flour Waffles with Berries and Crème Fraîche (page 58)	Roasted Leg of Lamb with Rice (page 118), steamed carrots and spinach, Fresh Berry and Cardamom Meringues (page 166)	Minty Melon Breakfast Juice (page 63) and Aubergine Dip with corn chips (page 75)	
MONDAY	Raspberry and Oatmeal Smoothie (page 61), slice of wheat-free toast with peanut butter	Cream of Courgette Soup (page 67)	Beef, Carrot and Squash (page 113) served with quinoa/buckwheat	Wheat-free cookies
TUESDAY	Scrambled eggs on wheat-free toast	Mini Baked Potatoes with Blue Cheese (page 137) and a green salad	Spiced Halibut Curry with basmati rice (page 98)	Fewer than 10 dried banana chips
WEDNESDAY	Multigrain Cereal (page 48) served with low-lactose milk and banana	Quinoa/rice salad with feta, corn, spinach, pine nuts and French dressing	Chicken with Spicy Red Pepper Sauce (page 110) and new potatoes	Corn chips
THURSDAY	Poached egg, a rasher (strip) of bacon and slice of wheat-free toast	Courgette and Feta Fritters (page 131)	Pork and Cranberry Meatloaf (page 122) served with spring greens and new potatoes	Italian Rice Cake (page 171)
FRIDAY	Bubble and Squeak (page 52) using leftover spring greens/potatoes	Roasted Pumpkin Soup (page 68) with rice/oatcakes	Scallops with Bacon and Sage (page 103) with steamed buckwheat/quinoa, Chocolate Espresso Mousse (page 165)	Handful raisins/sultanas (golden raisins)

TWO-WEEK LOW-FODMAP VEGETARIAN PLAN

	BREAKFAST/BRUNCH	LUNCH	SUPPER	SNACKS
SATURDAY	Cheese Cornbread Muffins (page 57) – replace bacon with 50g/2oz pine nuts	Cream of Courgette Soup (page 67)	Thai Yellow Vegetable Curry (page 126) served with rice/buckwheat, if desired	Small handful dried fruit and almonds
SUNDAY	Quinoa Frittata (page 55) – omit salmon	Aubergine Dip (page 75) served with rice cakes and cucumber	Stuffed Courgettes (page 134) served with baked potato wedges	Polenta Cake (page 170)
MONDAY	Granola (page 49) served with 30ml/ 2 tbsp Greek (strained plain) yogurt	Egg mayonnaise sandwich (made with 2 slices of wheat-free bread)	Aubergine Pilaff with Cinnamon and Mint (page 128)	Courgette and Ginger Cake (page 172)
TUESDAY	Wheat-free toast with peanut butter or butter and yeast extract	Mini Baked Potatoes with Blue Cheese (page 137) and side salad	Corn Fritters (page 78) with stir-fried mixed (bell) peppers and green cabbage, Blueberry Parfait (page 162)	Fresh or canned pineapple slice
WEDNESDAY	Porridge made with low-lactose milk	Grated Cheddar and walnut salad (using suitable ingredients)	Egg, Potato and Green Pea Curry (page 127) with steamed rice	Soya yogurt
THURSDAY	30ml/2 tbsp Greek/ raspberry yogurt with sliced banana, Blueberry Muffin (page 60)	Fried egg, served with Spiced Potato Cakes (page 139)	Miso Broth with Tofu (page 72)	Olives
FRIDAY	Cornflakes/puffed rice with low-lactose milk and sliced strawberries	Radicchio Frittata (page 133)	Courgette and Feta Fritters (page 131) with side salad and mayonnaise, Baked Bananas with Toffee Sauce (page 155)	Rice cakes

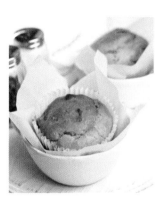
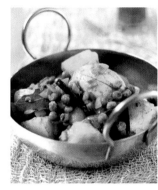
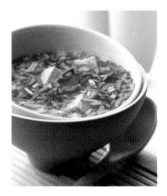

	BREAKFAST/BRUNCH	LUNCH	SUPPER	SNACKS
SATURDAY	Buckwheat Pancakes (page 56), served with sliced mozzarella or a poached egg	Rice salad (rice, peppers, tomatoes, cucumber, toasted pine nuts)	Aubergine Dip with corn chips (page 75), Mini Baked Potatoes and Blue Cheese (page 137)	2 squares milk chocolate
SUNDAY	Oat Flour Waffles with Berries and Crème Fraîche (page 58) with Minty Melon Breakfast Juice (page 63)	Cheese and spinach omelette served with Polenta Chips (page 79), side salad and mayonnaise, Fresh Berry and Cardamom Meringues (page 166)	Handful of peanuts	
MONDAY	Zesty Soya Smoothie (page 62), slice of wheat-free toast with peanut butter	Toasted Rice, Buckwheat and Corn Bread (page 173) with scrambled egg	Roasted Peppers with Halloumi and Pine Nuts (page 132)	Small glass orange juice
TUESDAY	Scrambled eggs on wheat-free toast	Fennel with Parmesan (page 140) and side salad	Jacket potato topped with feta cheese, sun-dried tomatoes and toasted slivered almonds	Raspberry Friands (page 169)
WEDNESDAY	Multigrain Cereal (page 48) served with low-lactose milk and banana	Lettuce and Egg Salad (page 145)	Wheat-free pasta served with Cheese Sauce (page 39) and steamed spinach	Few squares of plain (semi sweet) chocolate
THURSDAY	Boiled egg, wheat-free toast	Roasted Pumpkin Soup (page 68) with rice/oatcakes	Baked Aubergines with Mozzarella (page 141), with mashed potato and steamed spring greens	Fewer than 10 dried banana chips, rice cakes with cream cheese
FRIDAY	Bubble and Squeak (page 52) (made from last night's potato/spring greens)	Miso Broth with Tofu (page 72) with wheat-free crackers	Potato and Parsnip Gratin (page 136), Chocolate Espresso Mousse (page 165)	Sliced orange

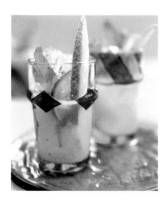
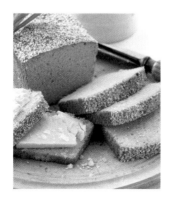
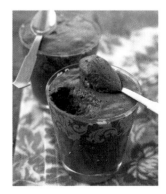

RE-INTRODUCTION FOOD DIARY

Scan or photocopy this diary and use it to record your daily FODMAP intake during the re-introduction phase. It is very important that you record any symptoms.

DAY	BREAKFAST	LUNCH	DINNER
SATURDAY			
SUNDAY			
MONDAY			
TUESDAY			
WEDNESDAY			
THURSDAY			
FRIDAY			
SATURDAY			
SUNDAY			
MONDAY			
TUESDAY			
WEDNESDAY			
THURSDAY			
FRIDAY			

DRINKS	SNACKS	SYMPTOMS

Introduction

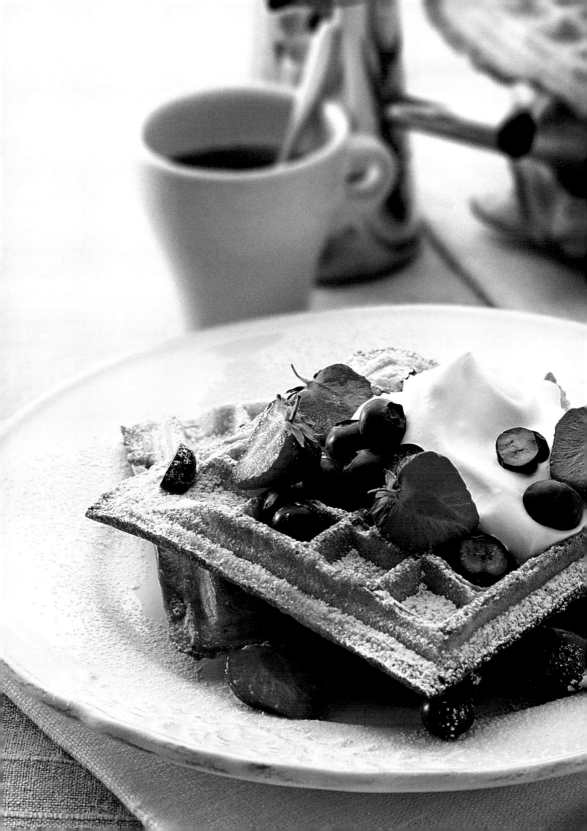

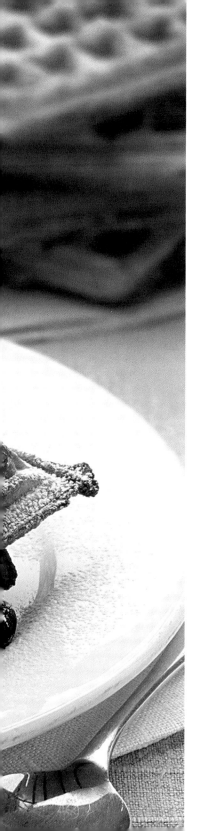

BREAKFASTS

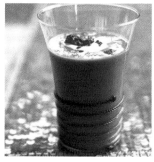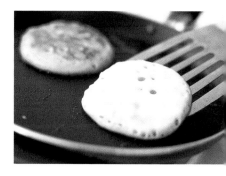

A little creative thinking will ensure that
your wheat-free, low-lactose breakfasts
don't become restrictive or repetitive. These
recipes use a range of healthy ways to start
your day with fruit, oats, seeds, nuts, fish,
eggs, and even bacon, that may leave you
wondering what you ate before!

MULTIGRAIN CEREAL

Although wheat-free cereal has now become much more easy to find, making your own is fun and allows you to tailor and vary it to your own tastes. Use extra crisped rice cereal, or cornflakes, if you can't find quinoa pops.

FODMAP TYPE: Lactose
NUTRITIONAL CONTENT:
Energy 254kcal/1062kJ;
Protein 7g; Carbohydrate 35g,
of which sugars 7g; Fat 11g, of
which saturates 1g; Cholesterol
0mg; Calcium 67mg; Fibre 2g;
Sodium 102mg

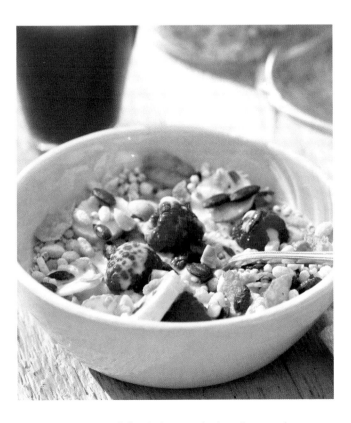

SERVES 6

50g/2oz/⅓ cup hazelnuts
50g/2oz/¼ cup pumpkin seeds
50g/2oz/½ cup rolled oats
25g/1oz/1 cup quinoa pops
50g/2oz/1 cup crisped rice
   cereal
25g/1oz/⅔ cup cornflakes
25g/1oz/⅙ cup dried
   blueberries
25g/1oz/⅙ cup dried
   cranberries
natural (plain) yogurt, maple
   syrup, lactose-free milk, or
   fresh fruit, to serve

COOK'S TIP Quinoa pops are puffed quinoa seeds. They are available in health stores and online.

VARIATION Use other low-FODMAP dried fruit and nuts if you wish. Pecans or almonds combine well with sunflower seeds.

Under a medium grill (broiler), toast the hazelnuts and pumpkin seeds for a few minutes until the seeds start to pop and the nuts are browning. Watch the nuts closely, as it is easy to scorch them.

Roughly crush the toasted hazelnuts with the end of a rolling pin. Set aside to cool completely. Mix the cooled nuts and seeds with the remaining ingredients in a large bowl and store in an airtight container.

Serve with lactose-free milk, or 30ml/2 tbsp natural yogurt. Add fresh fruit and maple syrup or sugar if desired.

GRANOLA

Dried fruit is high in the natural sugar, fructose, which is a FODMAP ingredient. However, limiting this to the correct amount per portion keeps the load manageable and shouldn't cause IBS symptoms in most people.

Preheat the oven to 140°C/275°F/Gas 1. Mix together the oats, seeds and nuts in a bowl.

Heat the oil and maple syrup in a large pan until melted, then remove the pan from the heat. Add the oat mixture and stir well. Spread out on one or two baking sheets.

Bake for about 50 minutes until crisp, stirring occasionally to prevent the mixture sticking.

Remove from the oven and mix in the raisins and cranberries. Leave to cool, then store in an airtight container.

FODMAP TYPE: Lactose
NUTRITIONAL CONTENT:
Energy 311kcal/1300kJ;
Protein 7g; Carbohydrate 32g,
of which sugars 9g; Fat 18g, of
which saturates 2g; Cholesterol
0mg; Calcium 66mg; Fibre 3g;
Sodium 14mg

SERVES 8

115g/4oz/1 cup rolled oats
115g/4oz/1 cup jumbo oats
50g/2oz/½ cup sunflower seeds
25g/1oz/2 tbsp sesame seeds
50g/2oz/½ cup hazelnuts,
  roasted
25g/1oz/¼ cup almonds,
  roughly chopped
50ml/2fl oz/¼ cup sunflower oil
50ml/2fl oz/¼ cup maple syrup
25g/1oz/¼ cup raisins
25g/1oz/¼ cup dried sweetened
  cranberries

Breakfasts

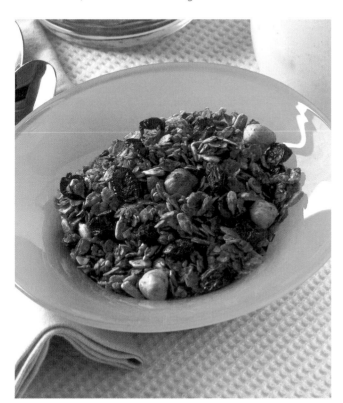

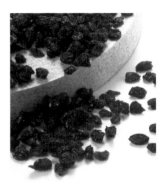

SMOKED SALMON BREAKFAST WRAPS

Some FODMAP foods, such as avocado and cream cheese, are fine but only if served in controlled quantities. In this recipe, therefore, be careful to stick to the amounts and serving quantity.

FODMAP TYPE: Lactose
NUTRITIONAL CONTENT:
Energy 401kcal/1676kJ;
Protein 12g; Carbohydrate 40g,
of which sugars 3g; Fat 22g, of
which saturates 8g; Cholesterol
25mg; Calcium 117mg; Fibre 3g;
Sodium 609mg

Breakfasts

SERVES 6

2 red (bell) peppers
30ml/2 tbsp olive oil
6 large wheat-free tortillas
1 avocado
30ml/2 tbsp lemon juice
115g/4oz/½ cup cream cheese
   mixed with 15ml/1 tbsp
   chopped fresh dill
25g/1oz/3 tbsp pine nuts
50g/2oz baby spinach leaves
115g/4oz smoked salmon
salt and ground black pepper
lemon wedges, to serve

Preheat the oven to 180°C/350°F/Gas 4. Place the peppers in a roasting pan. Drizzle the olive oil over and season with plenty of salt and black pepper. Bake for 25–30 minutes.

Peel the skin off the cooked peppers and discard the core and seeds. Cut the pepper flesh into strips.

Place the tortillas on a sheet of foil and seal tightly. Warm in the oven for 10 minutes.

Meanwhile, cut the avocado in half, remove the stone (pit) and peel, then slice lengthways. Sprinkle with the lemon juice to prevent the avocado flesh from turning brown.

Remove the tortillas from the oven. Spread a sixth of the cream cheese and dill over each wrap, then sprinkle the pine nuts evenly over the top, leaving the borders free.

Divide the avocado, spinach, salmon and peppers among the tortillas, placing them in a line down the centre. Roll up each wrap and serve immediately, while still warm. Offer lemon wedges for squeezing over.

VARIATION You could also use wheat-free pitta bread or taco shells in place of the tortillas.

COOK'S TIP For extra crunch and flavour try toasting the pine nuts in a small frying pan for a few minutes. Cool completely before adding to the wrap filling.

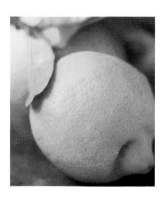

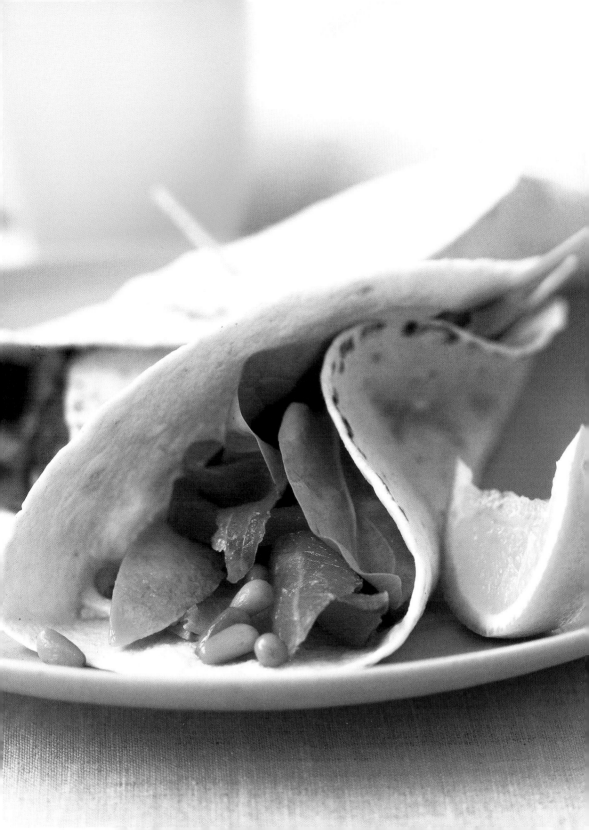

BUBBLE AND SQUEAK

Traditionally made from leftover vegetables, bubble and squeak can be made from whatever you have to hand. Try incorporating other cooked low-FODMAP vegetables such as spinach, white cabbage or carrots.

Breakfasts

FODMAP TYPE: Lactose
NUTRITIONAL CONTENT:
Energy 231kcal/966kJ;
Protein 12g; Carbohydrate 45g,
of which sugars 6g; Fat 2g, of
which saturates 0g; Cholesterol
0mg; Calcium 270mg; Fibre 11g;
Sodium 103mg

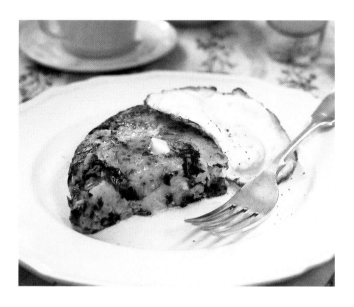

SERVES 2

60ml/4 tbsp oil
4 spring onions (scallions),
    green tops only, thinly sliced
450g/1lb cooked, mashed
    potatoes
225g/8oz cooked spring greens,
    chopped
salt and ground black pepper
2 fried eggs, to serve

VARIATION Bubble and squeak also makes a quick and easy supper, when you could use garlic-infused olive oil for added flavour.

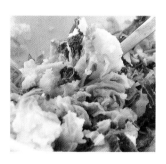

Heat half the oil in a heavy, preferably non-stick frying pan. Add the chopped spring onion greens and cook, stirring until softened but not browned.

Mix together the cooked mashed potatoes and spring greens and season to taste with salt and plenty of pepper. Add the vegetable mixture to the pan, stir to incorporate, then flatten out over the base of the pan to form a large, even cake.

Cook over a medium heat for about 15 minutes, until the cake is nicely browned underneath.

Hold a large plate over the pan, then invert the cake onto it. Add the remaining oil to the pan and, when hot, slip the cake back into the pan, browned side uppermost.

Continue cooking for about 10 minutes, until the underside is golden brown. Serve hot, cut into wedges with a fried egg.

SMOKED HADDOCK AND CHEESE OMELETTE

This winning protein-rich breakfast combination will set you up well for a productive day. Full-fat cream and hard cheese are both low in FODMAP lactose, so are fine to use in these quantities.

Remove and discard the skin and any bones from the haddock fillet. Using two forks and following the grain of the flesh, flake the fish into large chunks.

Melt half the butter with 60ml/4 tbsp of the cream in a small pan. When the mixture is hot but not boiling, add the fish. Cover the pan, remove from the heat and set aside for at least 20 minutes.

Preheat the grill (broiler) to high. Stir the egg yolks into the fish and season with black pepper. In a separate bowl, mix the cheese and the remaining cream. Stiffly whisk the egg whites, then fold into the fish mixture.

Heat the remaining butter in an omelette pan until foaming. Add the fish mixture and cook until it is browned underneath. Pour the cheese mixture evenly over the top and grill (broil) until bubbling. Serve straight away.

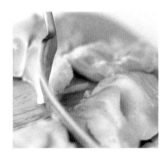

Breakfasts

SERVES 2

175g/6oz smoked haddock
   fillet
50g/2oz butter, diced
75ml/2½fl oz/⅓ cup whipping
   or double (heavy) cream
4 eggs, separated
40g/1½oz mature (sharp)
   Cheddar cheese, grated
ground black pepper

COOK'S TIP Whisking the egg whites gives the omelette its fluffiness. If you are short of time add the yolks and whites together.

FODMAP TYPE: Lactose
NUTRITIONAL CONTENT:
Energy 608kcal/2541kJ;
Protein 35g; Carbohydrate 1g,
of which sugars 1g; Fat 52g, of
which saturates 28g; Cholesterol
525mg; Calcium 247mg; Fibre
0g; Sodium 1033mg

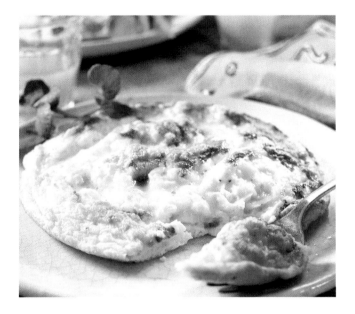

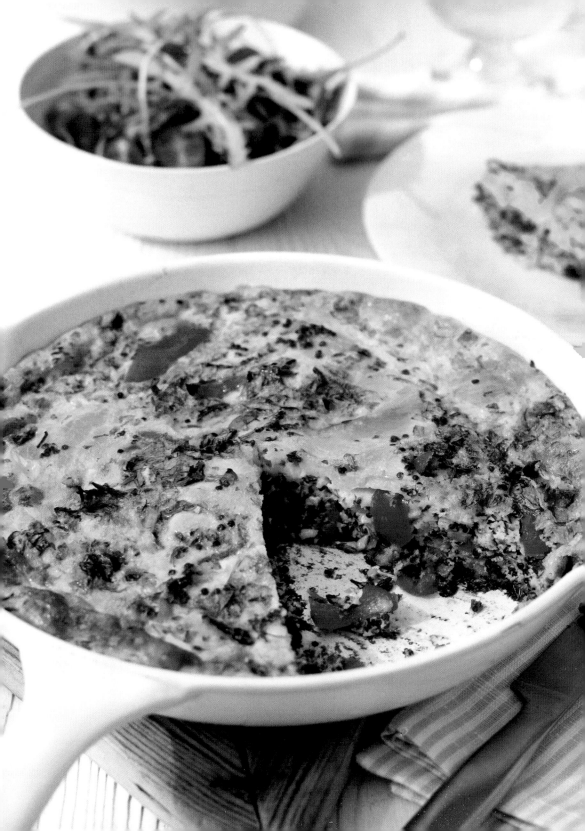

SALMON AND QUINOA FRITTATA

Quinoa is a highly nutritious wheat-free seed, grown for centuries in the Andes mountains of South America. It is rich in protein, iron and calcium, and is also an excellent carbohydrate source on a low-FODMAP diet.

Heat the oil in a heavy frying pan or skillet and add the chopped pepper. Stir-fry for 8–10 minutes until soft, then add the fenugreek seeds, if using, and cook for 2 minutes.

Add the rocket and cook for a few more minutes until the leaves have wilted.

Meanwhile, whisk together the crème fraîche, beaten eggs, herbs and seasoning in a small bowl.

Add the salmon and quinoa to the frying pan, mix well, then spread evenly over the base of the pan.

Pour the beaten egg mixture into the pan, lower the heat, and cook for 5–8 minutes until the frittata is cooked most of the way through (you can test this by carefully pressing it with a fork). Covering the pan with a lid will help ensure even cooking. Heat the grill (broiler) to medium.

Sprinkle the grated cheese over the top of the frittata, then place under the grill, making sure the handle is not exposed to heat, for 3–5 minutes until the frittata is puffed and golden brown. Serve warm or at room temperature.

VARIATIONS Swap salmon for another oily fish such as mackerel, tuna or sardines, and replace the quinoa with rice or cooked, cubed potato.

FODMAP TYPE: Lactose
NUTRITIONAL CONTENT:
Energy 205kcal/857kJ;
Protein 15g; Carbohydrate 6g, of which sugars 2g; Fat 13g, of which saturates 5g; Cholesterol 214mg; Calcium 145mg; Fibre 1g; Sodium 447mg

SERVES 4

15ml/1 tbsp olive oil
1 orange or red (bell) pepper, chopped
5ml/1 tsp fenugreek seeds (optional)
75g/3oz rocket (arugula), roughly chopped
30ml/2 tbsp crème fraîche
6 eggs, beaten
a handful of parsley, finely chopped
100g/3¾oz smoked salmon, cut into thin strips
115g/4oz/⅔ cup cooked red quinoa
50g/2oz/½ cup grated strong cheese such as Emmenthal or Parmesan
salt and ground black pepper

Breakfasts

BUCKWHEAT PANCAKES WITH GRILLED BACON

Buckwheat is actually a fruit seed related to rhubarb and sorrel, and is an excellent wheat-free alternative, popular in Russia and Northern China. Its flour has a natural sweetness that lends itself to baking, particularly for pancakes.

FODMAP TYPE: lactose
NUTRITIONAL CONTENT:
Energy 297kcal/1241kJ;
Protein 11g; Carbohydrate 24g,
of which sugars 1g; Fat 17g, of
which saturates 7g; Cholesterol
84mg; Calcium 17mg; Fibre 2g;
Sodium 825mg

Breakfasts

SERVES 4

240ml/8fl oz/1 cup lactose-free
  milk, eg soya or rice
1 egg
2.5ml/½ tsp vanilla extract
130g/4½oz/1 cup buckwheat
  flour
5ml/1 tsp baking powder
5ml/1 tsp bicarbonate of soda
  (baking soda)
vegetable oil or butter, for
  frying
salt
butter, and 115g/4oz grilled
  (broiled) bacon (25g/1oz per
  person), to serve

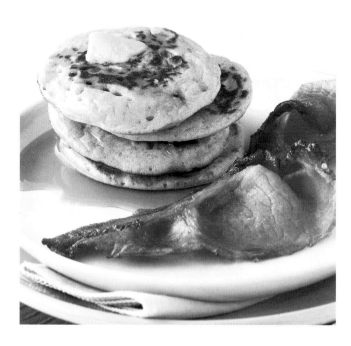

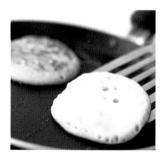

Whisk the milk with the egg in a small bowl and add the vanilla extract and a pinch of salt.

In a medium bowl, sift the flour, baking powder and bicarbonate of soda together. Make a well in the centre and add the egg mixture, whisking to incorporate, a little at a time, to make a smooth, thick batter.

In a non-stick pan, heat the oil or butter. Add spoonfuls of the batter, a few at a time, to make approximately 8–12 pancakes about 6–7.5cm/2–3in in diameter. Flip over halfway through cooking to cook the other side. When golden, remove from the pan and keep warm until all the batter is used up.

To serve, spread the pancakes with a little butter, and serve with a piece of crispy, grilled bacon on the side.

BACON AND CHEESE CORNBREAD MUFFINS

Cornmeal is made from dried corn kernels and can be of variable coarseness. Finely ground it is also known as polenta, though that is actually the Italian dish made from cornmeal. These low-FODMAP muffins are portable and sustaining.

Heat the oven to 200°C/400°F/Gas 6. In a medium bowl, whisk together the yogurt with the eggs and oil.

Sift the polenta and baking powder into a large bowl, and mix in the grated cheese and diced bacon. Make a well in the middle and add the yogurt mixture, and quickly mix together.

Divide the mixture between 12 muffin cases in a muffin tin or pan, and bake for approximately 20 minutes until risen, golden and firm to touch. Cool on a wire rack for 12–15 minutes and eat warm, or cool completely and store in an airtight container.

COOK'S TIP Make sure that the bacon is finely diced to ensure that it cooks through.

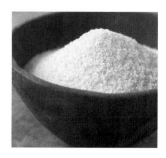

240ml/8fl oz/1 cup natural (plain) yogurt
2 eggs
90ml/6 tbsp olive oil
225g/8oz/1½ cups fine cornmeal/polenta
15ml/1 tbsp baking powder
85g/3oz grated cheese
85g/3oz lean, smoked, bacon rashers (strips), finely diced

VARIATION Add a handful of corn for a muffin with extra bite and fibre.

FODMAP TYPE: Lactose
NUTRITIONAL CONTENT:
Energy 185kcal/773kJ;
Protein 7g; Carbohydrate 16g, of which sugars 2g; Fat 10g, of which saturates 3g; Cholesterol 42mg; Calcium 95mg; Fibre 1g; Sodium 180mg

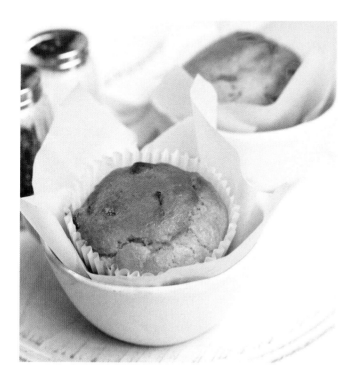

OAT FLOUR WAFFLES WITH BERRIES AND CRÈME FRAÎCHE

Oats are rich in soluble fibre, are also low-glycaemic index and are great for breakfast, as they will keep you satisfied for longer. Oat flour can be made easily at home. You will need a waffle maker or pan for this recipe.

FODMAP TYPE: Lactose
NUTRITIONAL CONTENT:
Energy 239kcal/999kJ;
Protein 6g; Carbohydrate 21g,
of which sugars 2g; Fat 15g, of
which saturates 8g; Cholesterol
93mg; Calcium 30mg; Fibre 2g;
Sodium 121mg

Breakfasts

SERVES 4–6

140g/5oz/1½ cups rolled oats or
    wholegrain oat flour
80g/3oz/⅓ cup butter, plus
    5ml/1 tsp for greasing
2 eggs
180ml/6fl oz/¾ cup lactose-free
    milk, eg soya or rice
5ml/1 tsp baking powder
a handful of low-FODMAP
    berries eg blueberries,
    strawberries, raspberries,
    maple syrup and crème
    fraîche, or natural (plain)
    yogurt, to serve
icing (confectioners') sugar,
    for dusting

Make the oat flour by grinding the oats in a food processor or blender until coarse, or finer if you prefer. You could do this in a pestle and mortar too.

In a pan on the hob, or in a microwaveable dish, soften the butter. Beat in the eggs, one at a time, then add the milk alternative, and whisk until smooth.

Tip the oat flour into a bowl and mix in the baking powder. Make a well in the middle, then add the egg and milk mixture. Gradually pull the flour into the milk and egg until it is all incorporated, and a smooth batter is formed.

Heat up the waffle maker or stove iron, grease with the extra butter, and then add the waffle batter, cooking until puffed and golden.

Serve warm with berries, syrup and crème fraîche, dusted with icing sugar. The waffles will also keep in an airtight container when cooled, and can be reheated later.

COOK'S TIP You can make the batter in advance and store in the refrigerator covered for up to 48 hours. Remember to avoid fructose-rich honey or agave syrup when serving.

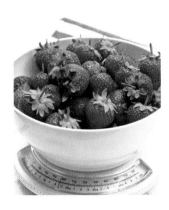
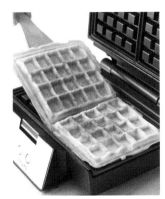

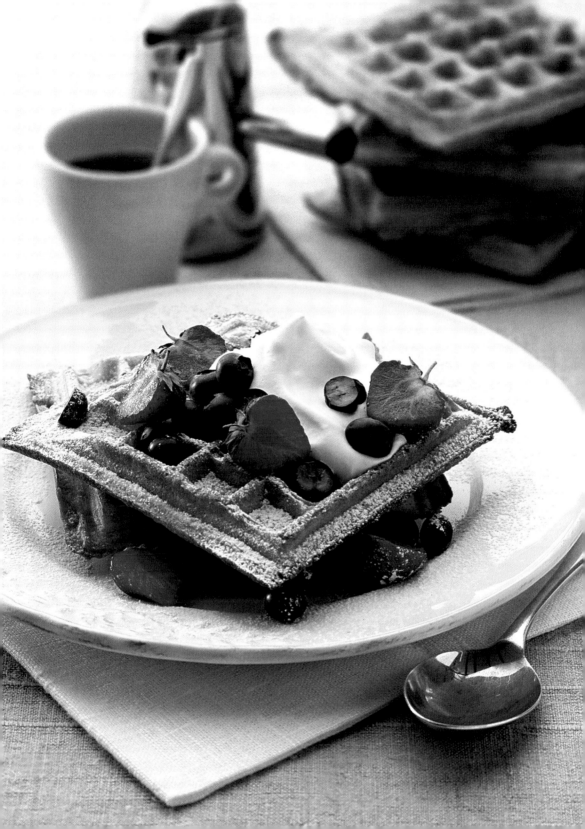

BLUEBERRY MUFFINS

Pale yellow maize flour tends to be higher in fat, protein and fibre than cornmeal as the whole kernel is milled. Like the cornbread muffins, these sweet alternatives are perfect served warm, or as a low-FODMAP snack on the move.

FODMAP TYPE: Lactose
NUTRITIONAL CONTENT:
Energy 178kcal/744kJ;
Protein 4g; Carbohydrate 26g,
of which sugars 8g; Fat 7g, of
which saturates 4g; Cholesterol
46mg; Calcium 12mg; Fibre 1g;
Sodium 59mg

Breakfasts

MAKES 12

175ml/6fl oz/¾ cup lactose-free
    milk, eg soya or rice
2 eggs
75g/3oz butter, melted
275g/10oz/1¼ cups maize flour
15ml/1 tbsp baking powder
75g/3oz/1 cup soft light brown
    sugar
115g/4oz fresh or frozen
    blueberries

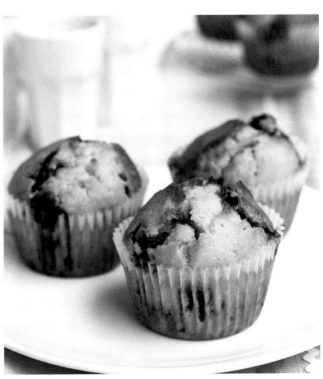

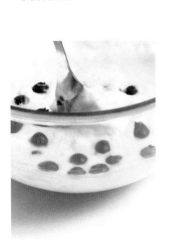

Heat the oven to 200°C/400°F/Gas 6. In a medium bowl, whisk together the milk and the eggs, then mix in the melted butter.

In a large bowl sift the flour and baking powder, then mix in the sugar. Add the milk mixture and combine, then stir in the blueberries. Don't over-mix.

Divide the mixture between 12 muffin cases inside a muffin tin or pan. Bake for approximately 20 minutes until risen, golden and firm to touch.

Cool on a wire rack for 12–15 minutes, then eat warm, or cool completely and store in an airtight container.

RASPBERRY AND OATMEAL SMOOTHIE

Ground oats (oatmeal) are wheat- and FODMAP- free, and are also rich in sustaining soluble fibre that helps lower blood cholesterol levels. Make this smoothie in advance, using a portable container, for breakfast on the go.

Spoon the oatmeal into a heatproof bowl. Pour in 120ml/ 4fl oz/½ cup boiling water and leave to stand for 10 minutes.

Put the soaked oats in a food processor or blender and add the raspberries, maple syrup and about 30ml/2 tbsp of the crème fraîche. Whizz until smooth and creamy.

Pour the raspberry and oatmeal smoothie into a large glass, swirl in the remaining crème fraîche and top with a few extra raspberries.

FODMAP TYPE: Lactose
NUTRITIONAL CONTENT:
Energy 140kcal/585kJ;
Protein 3g; Carbohydrate 13g;
of which sugars 6g; Fat 9g, of
which saturates 6g; Cholesterol
23mg; Calcium 36mg; Fibre 5g;
Sodium 10mg

SERVES 1

22.5ml/1½ tbsp medium
  oatmeal
150g/5oz/scant 1 cup
  raspberries
5–10ml/1–2 tsp maple syrup
45ml/3 tbsp crème fraîche
a few extra raspberries,
  to decorate

Breakfasts

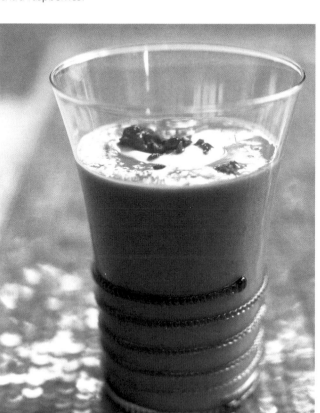

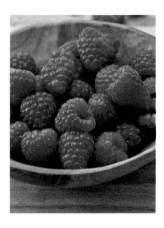

ZESTY SOYA SMOOTHIE

Tofu forms the basis of this refreshing yet sustaining smoothie, which although it is made from soya beans is not high in FODMAPs. Eat with a slice of wheat-free toast for a perfectly-balanced start to the day.

FODMAP TYPE: Lactose
NUTRITIONAL CONTENT:
Energy 342kcal/1430kJ;
Protein 22g; Carbohydrate 45g;
of which sugars 42g; Fat 9g, of
which saturates 2g; Cholesterol
0mg; Calcium 693mg; Fibre 6g;
Sodium 20mg

Finely grate the rind of one orange and set aside. Use a citrus juicer to juice both oranges and pour the juice into a food processor or blender. Add the grated orange rind, lemon juice, maple syrup and tofu.

Whizz the ingredients until smooth and creamy, then pour into a glass. Decorate with the pared orange rind and serve.

COOK'S TIP This smoothie keeps well in the refrigerator, and can also be frozen.

Breakfasts

SERVES 1

2 oranges
15ml/1 tbsp lemon juice
20–25ml/4–5 tsp maple syrup,
    or to taste
150g/5oz silken tofu
long, thin strip of pared orange
    rind, to decorate

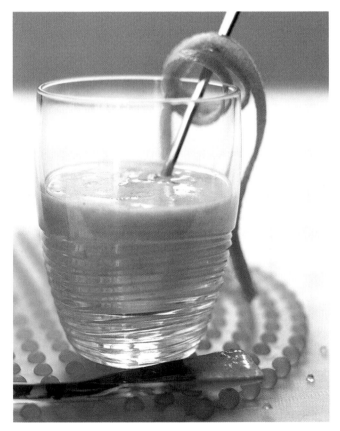

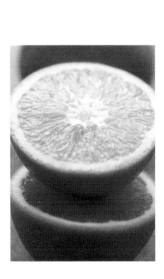

MINTY MELON BREAKFAST JUICE

Some melons, particularly watermelon and honeydew melon, are high in the FODMAP fructose, so don't be tempted to substitute either of these in this breakfast juice recipe. Perfect served with an oaty waffle or blueberry muffin.

Halve and seed the melon and cut into wedges. Cut one wedge into long, thin slices and reserve for decoration.

Cut the skin from the remaining wedges and push half the melon through a juicer or in a blender. Strip the mint leaves, push them through, then juice or blend the remaining melon.

Stir in the lime juice and pour over ice cubes in glasses. Decorate with mint sprigs and lime slices. Add a slice of melon to each glass and serve immediately.

FODMAP TYPE: Lactose
NUTRITIONAL CONTENT:
Energy 122kcal/510kJ;
Protein 3g; Carbohydrate 28g, of which sugars 28g; Fat Trace, of which saturates 0g; Cholesterol 0mg; Calcium 67mg; Fibre 5g; Sodium 155mg

SERVES 1

Breakfasts

½ galia or cantaloupe melon
several large mint sprigs
juice of 1 large lime
ice cubes
extra mint sprigs and lime
   slices, to decorate

COOK'S TIP Eat the pulp from the juicer mixed in with some natural (plain) yogurt.

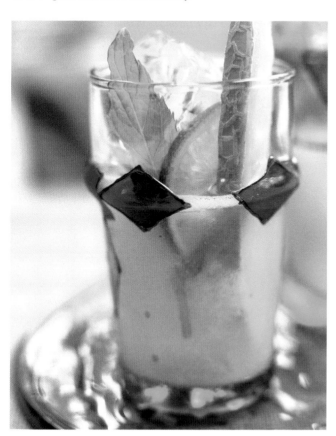

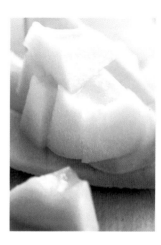

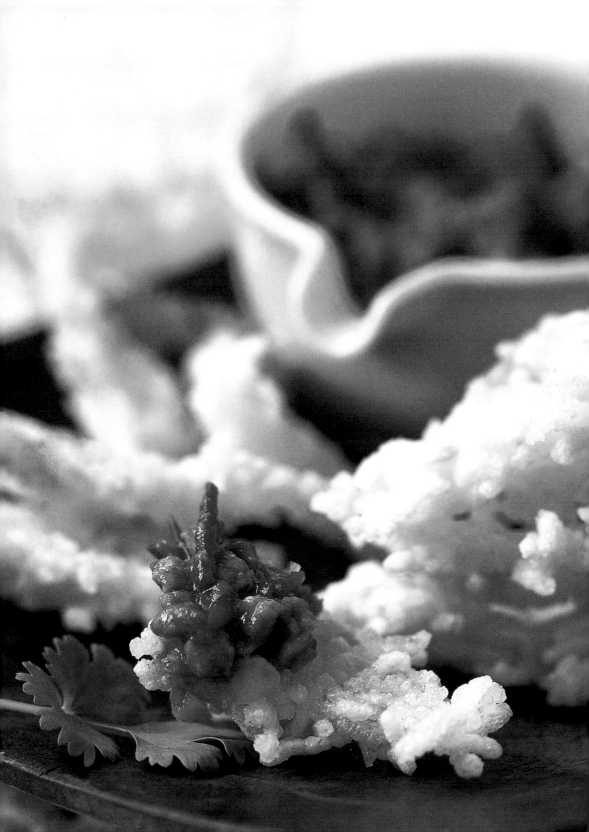

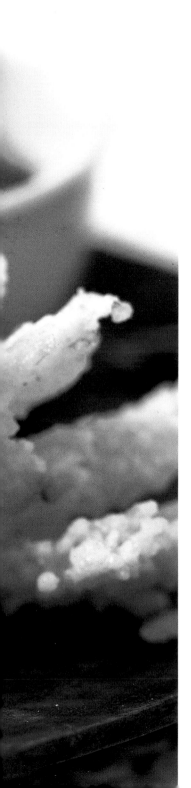

SOUPS, SNACKS & APPETIZERS

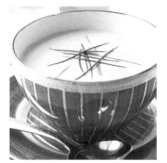 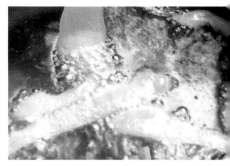

This chapter offers a range of soups, dips, fritters and crispy bites, which will give you inspiration for light meals or appetizers. Making use of FODMAP-friendly spices, herbs and chilli ensures that avoiding onion and garlic doesn't mean you have to compromise on taste or satisfaction.

CHICKEN AND LEMON SOUP

This simple Mediterranean recipe contains protein, zinc and vitamin-rich eggs in a chicken and lemon broth. However the chicken stock, whether homemade or fresh, should be free of FODMAP-rich onion and garlic.

FODMAP TYPE: Nil
NUTRITIONAL CONTENT:
Energy 79kcal/330kJ;
Protein 7g; Carbohydrate Trace,
of which sugars 0g; Fat 6g of
which saturates 2g; Cholesterol
193mg; Calcium 31mg; Fibre 0g;
Sodium 351mg

SERVES 4

1.2 litres/2 pints/5 cups fresh,
    low-FODMAP chicken stock
4 large eggs
juice of 2 large lemons
salt and ground black pepper
fresh chives, to garnish

COOK'S TIP This traditional Greek recipe must be made with the best-quality fresh chicken stock.

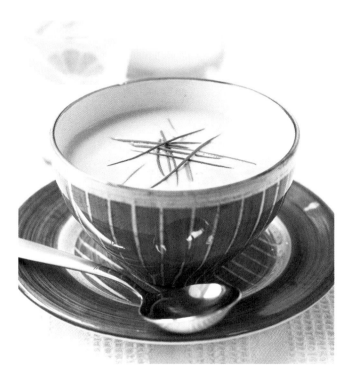

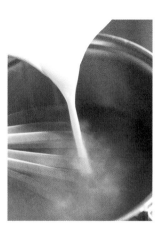

Pour the chicken stock into a large pan and bring it slowly to the boil. Meanwhile, break the eggs into a separate bowl and thoroughly whisk in the lemon juice.

Allow the stock to cool very slightly, then whisk a ladle-full of stock into the egg and lemon mixture.

Pour the lemon and egg mixture back into the pan of stock and cook over a very low heat, stirring continuously, until the soup is slightly thickened. Do not let the mixture boil.

Taste the soup and season lightly if required, then ladle into warmed bowls. Cut the chives into short lengths and scatter a few pieces on top of each portion. Serve immediately.

CREAM OF COURGETTE SOUP

Both cream and Dolcelatte contain some milk sugar, lactose, but many IBS sufferers are not affected by this in smaller amounts. If you do prefer to avoid lactose, or have an intolerance, use lactose-free alternatives.

Heat the oil and butter in a large pan until foaming. Add the courgettes and oregano, and season with salt and pepper. Cook over a medium heat for 10 minutes, stirring frequently.

When the courgettes are beginning to soften, pour in the stock and bring to the boil, stirring. Lower the heat, half cover the pan and simmer gently, stirring occasionally, for about 30 minutes. Stir in the diced Dolcelatte until melted.

Process in a blender or food processor until smooth. Press through a sieve or strainer into a clean pan. Add two-thirds of the cream and stir over a low heat until hot, but not boiling. Add a little more stock if the soup is too thick.

Taste for seasoning, then pour the soup into heated bowls. Swirl in the remaining cream. Garnish with oregano and extra cheese and serve.

FODMAP TYPE: Lactose
NUTRITIONAL CONTENT:
Energy 272kcal/1122kJ;
Protein 9g; Carbohydrate 6g, of which sugars 5g; Fat 23g, of which saturates 12g; Cholesterol 50mg; Calcium 197mg; Fibre 2g; Sodium 333mg

SERVES 4–6

30ml/2 tbsp olive oil
15g/½oz/1 tbsp butter
900g/2lb courgettes (zucchini), trimmed and sliced
5ml/1 tsp dried oregano
about 600ml/1 pint/2½ cups low-FODMAP chicken stock
115g/4oz Dolcelatte cheese, rind removed, diced
300ml/½ pint/1¼ cups single (light) cream
salt and ground black pepper
fresh oregano and extra Dolcelatte, to garnish

VARIATION This recipe would also work very well if you used parsnips instead of the courgettes.

Soups, Snacks & Appetizers

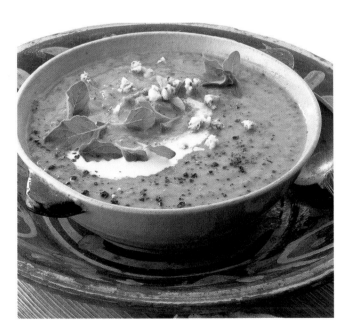

ROASTED PUMPKIN SOUP

Fortunately many herbs and spices are FODMAP friendly, which gives plenty of scope for creative cooking, in spite of the ban on onion and garlic. This recipe avoids having to peel and chop raw pumpkin, which can be time consuming.

FODMAP TYPE: Polyol (Mannitol)
NUTRITIONAL CONTENT:
Energy 54kcal/226kJ; Protein 3g; Carbohydrate 6g, of which sugars 4g; Fat 2g, of which saturates Trace; Cholesterol 0mg; Calcium 101mg; Fibre 3g; Sodium 143mg

SERVES 6

1.5kg/3–3½lb pumpkin
90ml/6 tbsp olive oil
7.5cm/3in piece fresh root ginger, grated
5ml/1 tsp ground coriander
2.5ml/½ tsp ground turmeric
pinch of cayenne pepper
1 litre/1¾ pints/4 cups vegetable stock
salt and ground black pepper
15ml/1 tbsp sesame seeds and fresh coriander (cilantro) leaves, to garnish

For the pumpkin crisps
wedge of fresh pumpkin, seeded
120ml/4fl oz/½ cup olive oil

COOK'S TIP Take care when cutting the roasted pumpkin as there may still be a lot of hot steam inside.

Preheat the oven to 200°C/400°F/Gas 6. Prick the pumpkin around the top several times with a fork, brush with plenty of oil and bake for 45 minutes or until tender. Leave to cool.

When cool enough to handle, cut the pumpkin in half and scoop out and discard the seeds. Scoop out and chop the flesh.

Heat about 60ml/4 tbsp of the remaining oil (you may not have to use all of it) in a large pan and add the ginger, stir for a few seconds to release the aroma, then add the coriander, turmeric and cayenne, and cook for 1 minute.

Add the pumpkin flesh and stock to the pan. Bring to the boil, reduce the heat and simmer for 20 minutes. Purée the soup in a food processor or blender until smooth, return to a clean pan and season.

Meanwhile, prepare the pumpkin crisps. Using a swivel-blade vegetable peeler, pare long thin strips from the wedge of pumpkin. Heat the oil in a small pan and fry the strips in batches for 2–3 minutes, until crisp. Drain on kitchen paper.

Reheat the soup and serve in bowls, topped with pumpkin crisps, sesame seeds and coriander leaves.

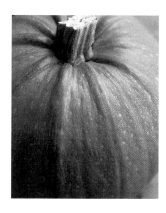
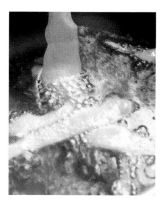

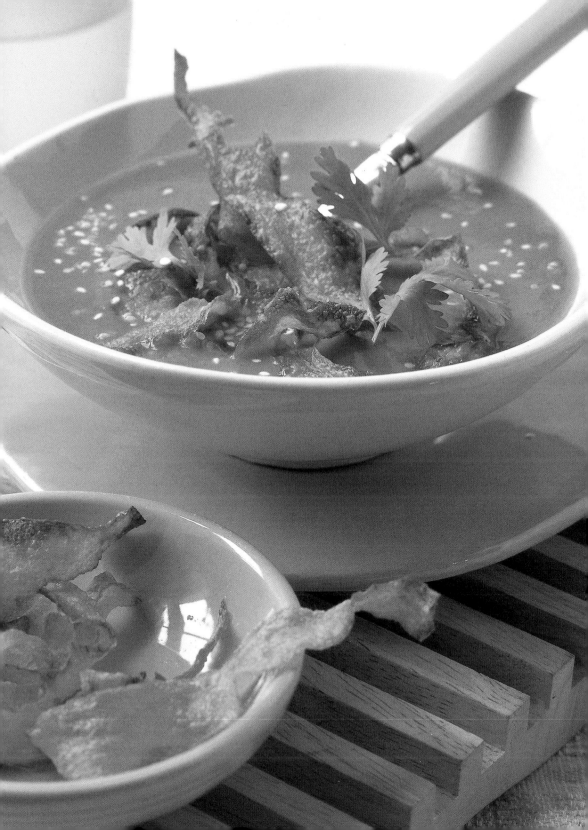

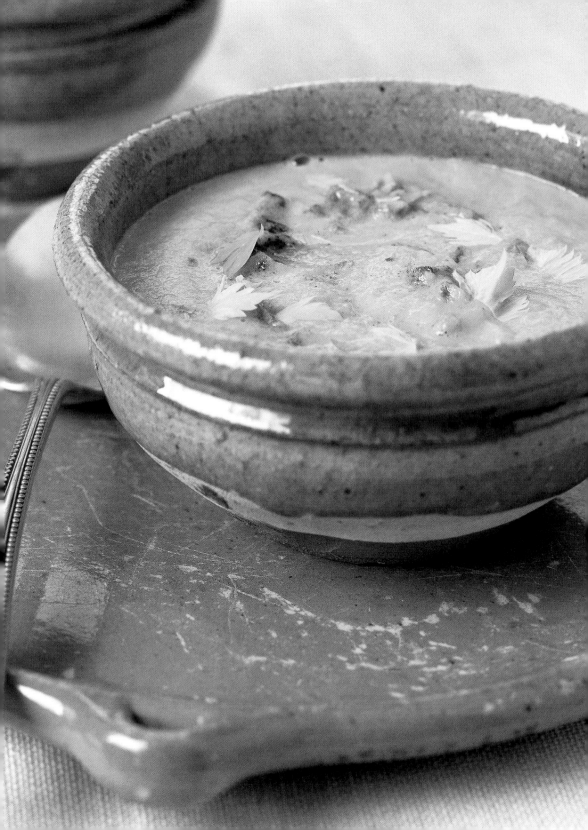

CARROT AND CORIANDER SOUP

Most root vegetables, with the exception of onion and garlic, are low FODMAP, and are ideal for bulking out classic winter warmers like this fabulous soup. Serve with wheat-free rolls for extra sustaining carbohydrates.

Slice the celery stick, reserving the leaves, and dice the peeled potatoes. Heat the oil and 25g/1oz/2 tbsp of the butter in a large pan and fry the sliced celery over a gentle heat for 3–4 minutes until slightly softened. Do not let it brown.

Add the diced potato and cook for 2 minutes, then add the carrots and cook for a further 1 minute.

Add the vegetable stock to the pan, then season with salt and ground black pepper. Cover the pot with the lid and simmer for 30–40 minutes until the vegetables are soft and tender.

Melt the remaining butter in a large pan and add the ground coriander. Fry for about 1 minute, stirring constantly, until the aromas are released, then add the fresh coriander. Fry for about 30 seconds, then remove the pan from the heat.

Ladle the soup into a food processor or blender and process until smooth, then pour into a clean pan and stir in the spice mixture. Add the cream and heat gently until piping hot.

Check the seasoning, then serve garnished with the reserved celery leaves.

FODMAP TYPE: Mannitol
NUTRITIONAL CONTENT:
Energy 196kcal/819kJ;
Protein 2g; Carbohydrate 15g,
of which sugars 9g; Fat 15g, of
which saturates 8g; Cholesterol
29mg; Calcium 51mg; Fibre 3g;
Sodium 309mg

SERVES 4	71

15ml/1 tbsp sunflower oil
40g/1½oz/3 tbsp butter
1 stick celery, plus 2–3 pale leafy tops
2 small potatoes, peeled and diced
450g/1lb carrots, peeled and cut into chunks
1.2 litres/2 pints/5 cups low-FODMAP vegetable stock
10ml/2 tsp ground coriander
15ml/1 tbsp chopped fresh coriander (cilantro)
60ml/3 tbsp double (heavy) cream
salt and ground black pepper

Soups, Snacks & Appetizers

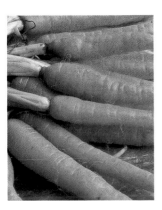
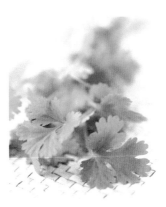

MISO BROTH WITH TOFU

Japanese miso paste is made from soya beans, which may contain traces of FODMAPs (GOS), but when processed into stock, miso is suitable for low-FODMAP cooking. Dashi no moto is stock made from fish and kelp so is also FODMAP friendly.

FODMAP TYPE: GOS
NUTRITIONAL CONTENT:
Energy 106kcal/443kJ;
Protein 10g; Carbohydrate 7g,
of which sugars 3g; Fat 4g, of
which saturates 5g; Cholesterol
0mg; Calcium 199mg; Fibre 1g;
Sodium 1590mg

SERVES 4

1 bunch of spring onions
    (scallions) green parts only,
    finely sliced
15g/½oz fresh coriander
    (cilantro), stalks and leaves
    separated, leaves finely
    chopped
3 thin slices fresh root ginger
2 star anise
1 small dried red chilli
1.2 litres/2 pints/5 cups dashi
    stock or low-FODMAP
    vegetable stock
225g/8oz pak choi (bok choy)
    or other greens, thinly sliced
200g/7oz firm tofu, cut into
    2.5cm/1in cubes
60ml/4 tbsp red miso
30–45ml/2–3 tbsp soy sauce
1 fresh red chilli, seeded and
    shredded (optional)

COOK'S TIP Tofu will fall apart as it is heated, so don't over-stir or boil too briskly.

Place the coriander stalks, fresh root ginger, star anise, dried chilli and dashi or vegetable stock in a large pan.

Heat the mixture gently until boiling, then lower the heat and simmer for 10 minutes. Strain, return to the pan and reheat. When simmering add the sliced spring onions and pak choi to the pan, together with the tofu. Cook for 2 minutes.

Mix 45ml/3 tbsp of the miso with a little of the hot soup in a bowl, then stir it into the soup. Add soy sauce to taste. Stir most of the chopped fresh coriander into the soup and cook for a further minute. Serve, sprinkled with the remaining coriander and fresh red chilli.

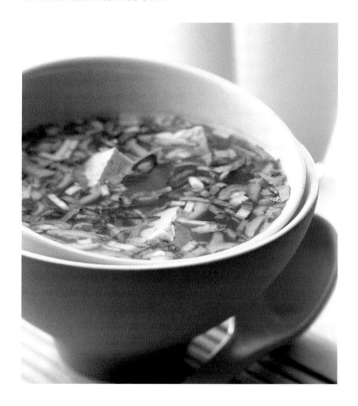

MISO SOUP WITH PORK

Protein staples of meat, fish, eggs and tofu are FODMAP-free, and here is another tasty oriental-style recipe, which makes use of low-FODMAP flavourings including miso and sesame. Serve with rice noodles for a more substantial supper.

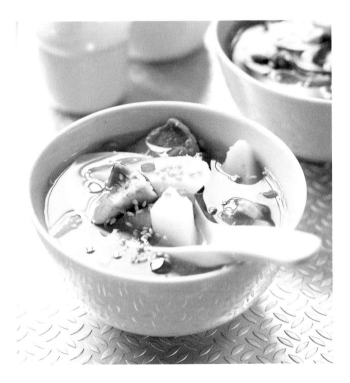

FODMAP TYPE: GOS
NUTRITIONAL CONTENT:
Energy 150kcal/627kJ;
Protein 18g; Carbohydrate 8g,
of which sugars 3g Fat 6g, of
which saturates 1g; Cholesterol
0mg; Calcium 133mg; Fibre 1g;
Sodium 812mg

SERVES 4

200g/7oz lean boneless pork,
  cut into thin strips
115g/4oz packet tofu
1 parsnip, peeled and sliced
50g/2oz water chestnuts sliced
a little sesame oil, for stir-frying
600ml/1 pint/2½ cups water
  mixed with 10ml/2 tsp dashi-
  no-moto
70ml/4½ tbsp miso
2 spring onions (scallions),
  green sections only, sliced
5ml/1 tsp sesame seeds

Soups, Snacks & Appetizers

Heat a little sesame oil in a large pan or wok until purple smoke rises. Stir-fry the pork, then add the tofu, and all the vegetables except for the spring onions. When the colour of the meat has changed, add the stock.

Bring to the boil over a medium heat, and skim off the foam until the soup looks fairly clear. Reduce the heat, cover, and simmer the stock for 15 minutes.

Put the miso in a small bowl, and mix with 60ml/4 tbsp hot stock to make a smooth paste. Stir one-third of the miso into the soup. Taste and add more miso if required. Add the sliced spring onion and remove from the heat. Serve very hot in individual soup bowls and sprinkle with sesame seeds.

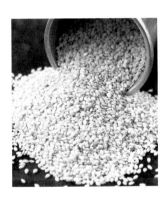

TAPENADE WITH QUAIL EGGS AND CRUDITÉS

This traditional Italian appetizer is bound to impress, but is very easy to put together. If you prefer to be completely lactose-free, omit the crème fraîche, and add a little more olive oil.

Soups, Snacks & Appetizers

FODMAP TYPE: Lactose
NUTRITIONAL CONTENT:
Energy 239kcal/999kJ; Protein 11g Carbohydrate Trace, of which sugars 0g; Fat 21g, of which saturates 5g; Cholesterol 679mg; Calcium 97mg; Fibre 2g Sodium 1078mg

74

SERVES 6

225g/8oz/2 cups pitted black olives
15ml/1 tbsp capers
6 anchovy fillets
50g/2oz canned tuna
5ml/1 tsp chopped fresh thyme
30ml/2 tbsp chopped fresh parsley
60ml/4 tbsp olive oil
a dash of lemon juice
30ml/2 tbsp crème fraîche
18 quail's eggs
salt and black pepper
radishes, sliced fennel or other raw vegetables to serve

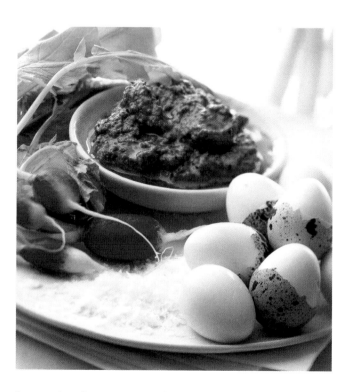

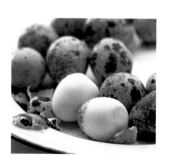

Process the olives, capers, anchovies and tuna in a food processor or blender. Blend in the thyme, parsley and enough olive oil to make a paste.

Season to taste with pepper and a dash of lemon juice. Stir in the crème fraîche, and transfer to a serving bowl.

Place the quail's eggs in a pan, cover with cold water and bring to the boil. Cook for only 2 minutes, then immediately drain and plunge the eggs into iced water to stop them from cooking further and to make them easier to shell.

Part-shell the cooled quail's eggs. Arrange the tapenade with the eggs and crudités and serve with sea salt.

AUBERGINE DIP

Unlike some nuts, such as pistachios and cashews, walnuts are fine as part of a low-FODMAP diet. Serve this tasty aubergine dip from Romania with wheat-free toasted pitta, or corn chips.

Spear the aubergines with a long-handled fork, or grip with tongs, and hold above the flame of a gas ring, or above an electric plate, turning until the aubergine is charred and soft.

Put the charred aubergines in a colander and leave them to cool. When cool enough to handle, peel off the blackened skin and discard. Squeeze the excess water out of the aubergines. Chop the flesh and put into a large bowl.

Add the lemon juice, olive oil and salt and pepper to taste, mix well and adjust the seasoning. Sprinkle with the parsley and walnuts. Serve cold.

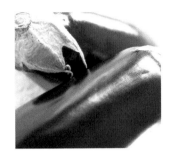

2 large aubergines (eggplants)
juice of 2 lemons
60ml/4 tbsp olive oil
75ml/5 tbsp chopped fresh
    parsley
50g/2oz/⅓ cup walnuts,
    coarsely chopped
salt and ground black pepper

COOK'S TIP Charring the aubergine gives a lovely smoky flavour, but you can also roast it whole in a high oven for a similar texture.

FODMAP TYPE: GOS, Fructans
NUTRITIONAL CONTENT:
Energy 111kcal/464kJ;
Protein 4g; Carbohydrate 4g;
of which sugars 3g; Fat 9g, of
which saturates 1g; Cholesterol
0mg; Calcium 55mg; Fibre 4g;
Sodium 301mg

Soups, Snacks & Appetizers

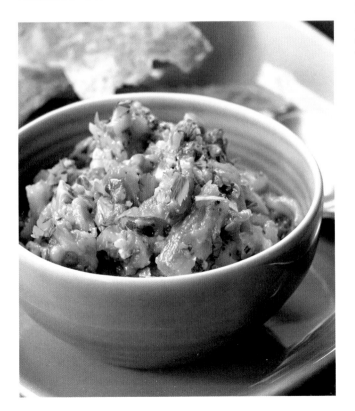

VEGETABLE TEMPURA

Crisp peppers and flavourful aubergine are perfect FODMAP-free vegetables for these mouthwatering morsels, but you could also use carrot or courgette, and smaller amounts of butternut squash and sweet potato.

FODMAP TYPE: Nil
NUTRITIONAL CONTENT:
Energy 286kcal/1195kJ;
Protein 5g; Carbohydrate 61g,
of which sugars 3g; Fat 4g, of
which saturates 1g; Cholesterol
98mg; Calcium 58mg; Fibre 3g;
Sodium 340mg

Soups, Snacks & Appetizers

SERVES 4

2 aubergines (eggplants), sliced
 into thin batons
2 red (bell) peppers, deseeded
 and thinly sliced
vegetable oil, for deep-frying
Thai sweet chilli sauce (see
 page 38), for serving

For the tempura batter
250g/9oz/2¼ cups cornflour
 (cornstarch)
2 egg yolks
500ml/17fl oz/2¼ cups iced
 water
5ml/1 tsp salt

Make the batter. Set aside 30ml/2 tbsp of the cornflour. Put the egg yolks in a large bowl and beat in the iced water. Tip in the remaining cornflour with the salt and stir briefly together – the mixture should resemble thick pancake batter but not properly mixed. If it is too thick, add a little more iced water.

Pour the oil for deep-frying into a wok or deep-fryer and heat to 190°C/375°F or until a cube of bread, added to the oil, browns in about 30 seconds.

Pick up a small handful of aubergine batons and pepper slices, dust with the reserved cornflour, dip into the batter then drop into the hot oil, taking care as the oil will froth up.

Repeat to make two or three more batches of tempura, but do not cook any more than this at one time, or the oil may overflow.

Cook for 3–4 minutes, until golden and crisp all over, then lift them out with a metal basket or slotted spoon. Drain thoroughly on kitchen paper and keep hot.

Repeat until all the vegetables have been coated in batter and cooked. Serve immediately, with the sweet chilli sauce.

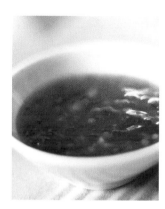
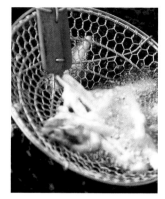

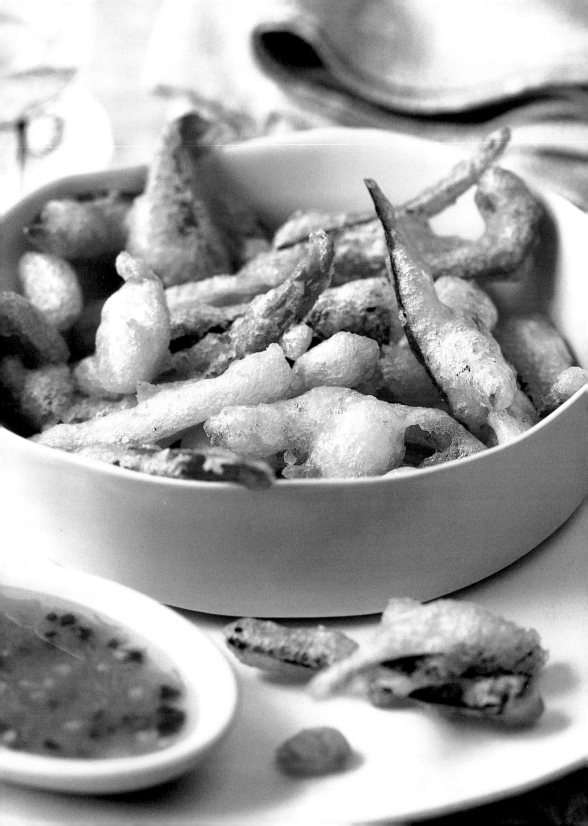

CORN FRITTERS

Corn should be limited to one cob per serving, which this recipe stays within, so long as fritters are limited to three per portion. However, this may prove a challenge once these deliciously crisp morsels are served.

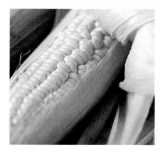

Using a sharp knife, slice the kernels from the cobs and place them in a large bowl. Add the chopped coriander, red or green chilli, spring onion, soy sauce, rice flour, beaten eggs and water and mix well. Season with salt and pepper. The mixture should be firm enough to hold its shape, but not stiff.

Heat the oil in a large frying pan. Add spoonfuls of the corn mixture, gently spreading each one out with the back of the spoon to make a roundish fritter. Cook for 1–2 minutes on each side.

Drain on kitchen paper and keep hot while frying more fritters in the same way. Serve hot with sweet chilli sauce.

Soups, Snacks & Appetizers

SERVES 4

3 corn on the cob
small bunch fresh coriander
    (cilantro), chopped
1 small fresh red or green chilli,
    seeded and finely chopped
1 spring onion (scallion), green
    part only, finely chopped
15ml/1 tbsp soy sauce
75g/3oz/¾ cup rice flour
2 eggs, lightly beaten
60ml/4 tbsp water
oil, for shallow frying
salt and ground black pepper
Thai sweet chilli sauce (see
    page 38), to serve

FODMAP TYPE: Sorbitol/Fructose
NUTRITIONAL CONTENT:
Energy 321kcal/1342kJ;
Protein 8g; Carbohydrate 32g,
of which sugars 3g; Fat 18g, of
which saturates 2g; Cholesterol
98mg; Calcium 29mg; Fibre 3g;
Sodium 306mg

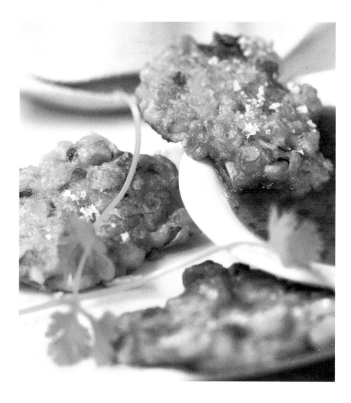

POLENTA CHIPS

Polenta is made with ground yellow or white cornmeal. Here it is allowed to set, then deep-fried, giving it a very moreish crunchy texture. These chips can be served with all sorts of dishes, or eaten as a snack with a cold beer.

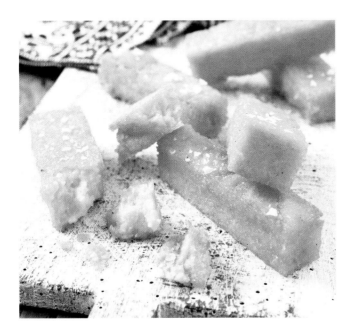

FODMAP TYPE: Nil
NUTRITIONAL CONTENT:
Energy 306kcal/1279kJ;
Protein 5g; Carbohydrate 46g,
of which sugars 0g; Fat 12g, of
which saturates 1g; Cholesterol
0mg; Calcium 2mg; Fibre 4g;
Sodium 157mg

SERVES 6

1 litre/1¾ pints/4¼ cups water
325g/12½oz/3¼ cups polenta
250ml/8fl oz/1 cup onion-free
  chicken stock
30ml/2 tbsp olive oil
30ml/2 tbsp cornflour
  (cornstarch)
vegetable oil, for deep-frying
coarse sea salt

Soups, Snacks & Appetizers

Pour the water into a large pan, add the polenta, stock and olive oil. Slowly bring to the boil, then simmer to a thick purée. The mixture is the correct consistency when the bottom of the pan starts to show as you stir. Sprinkle in the cornflour and continue cooking for another 3 minutes, stirring constantly.

Pour into an oiled 28 x 28cm/11 x 11in tin or pan, spreading in an even layer. Cool, then chill in the refrigerator for 1 hour to set.

Turn out the block of polenta on to a lightly oiled board. Wet the blade of a knife and use it to cut into 6cm/2½in long chips.

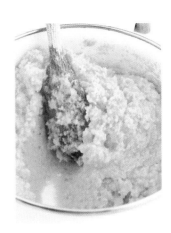

Half-fill a deep pan with oil, then heat to190°C/375°F. Add about a third of the chips, and fry for 3–4 minutes, until golden. Use a slotted spoon to remove them from the oil and drain on kitchen paper. Keep warm while cooking the remaining chips. Sprinkle with salt and serve straight away.

SALT AND PEPPER FRIED SQUID

Wheat-free flours work as well as their regular alternatives when coating foods for deep frying. Sourcing and preparing fresh squid is well worth the effort, but if not available using defrosted frozen fish will also be a treat.

FODMAP TYPE: Nil
NUTRITIONAL CONTENT:
Energy 249kcal/1041kJ;
Protein 18g; Carbohydrate 11g,
of which sugars 0g; Fat 14g, of
which saturates 1g; Cholesterol
25mg; Calcium 18mg; Fibre
Trace; Sodium 1652mg

SERVES 4

450g/1lb baby or medium squid
15ml/1 tbsp coarse salt
15ml/1 tbsp ground black
  pepper
50g/2oz/½ cup rice flour or
  cornflour (cornstarch)
vegetable oil, for frying
2 limes, halved

Prepare the squid by pulling the head away from the body. Sever the tentacles from the rest and trim them. Reach inside the body sac and pull out the backbone, then clean the squid inside and out, removing any skin. Rinse well in cold water.

Using a sharp knife, slice the squid into rings and pat them dry. Put them on a dish with the tentacles. Combine the salt and pepper with the rice flour or cornflour, tip it on to the squid and toss well, making sure it is evenly coated.

Heat the oil in a wok or heavy pan for deep-frying. Cook the squid in batches, until the rings turn crisp and golden. Drain on kitchen paper and serve with lime to squeeze over.

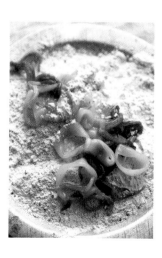

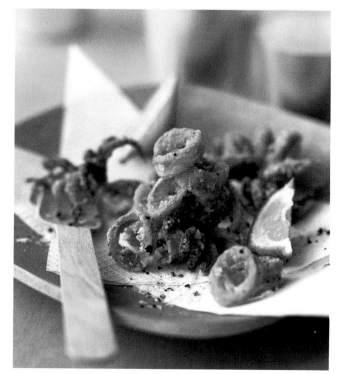

Soups, Snacks & Appetizers

FIERY SPICED CHICKEN WINGS WITH HARISSA

Add to the heat of a summer evening's barbecue with these tongue-tingling chicken wings. A recipe for FODMAP-free harissa paste can be found on page 37, it is really quick to make, and will keep in the refrigerator for a few weeks.

Put the harissa in a small bowl with the olive oil and mix to form a loose paste. Add a little salt and stir to combine. Brush this mixture over the chicken wings to coat completely.

Cook the wings on a hot barbecue or under a hot grill (broiler), for 5 minutes on each side, until golden and slightly charred.

While the wings are cooking, dip the orange quarters lightly in icing sugar and grill (broil) them for a few minutes, until they are slightly charred.

Serve the chicken wings immediately with the oranges, sprinkled with a little chopped fresh coriander.

FODMAP TYPE: Nil
NUTRITIONAL CONTENT:
Energy 455kcal/1902kJ; Protein 36g; Carbohydrate 19g, of which sugars 18g; Fat 27g, of which saturates 7g; Cholesterol 150mg; Calcium 131mg; Fibre 3g; Sodium 600mg

SERVES 4

60ml/4 tbsp harissa paste (see page 37)
30ml/2 tbsp olive oil
16–20 chicken wings
4 blood oranges, quartered
icing (confectioners') sugar, for dipping
small bunch of fresh coriander (cilantro), chopped
salt

Soups, Snacks & Appetizers

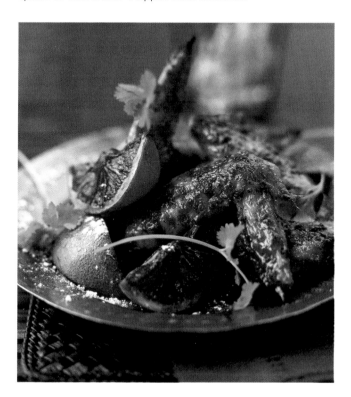

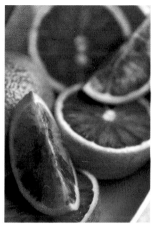

CRISPY RICE CAKES WITH SPICY DIP

You will need to plan ahead to prepare the rice cakes for this Thai treat, but the effort will be appreciated by your guests. Fresh coconut flesh is not FODMAP-free, but smaller amounts of coconut milk are luckily fine.

FODMAP TYPE: Sorbitol
NUTRITIONAL CONTENT:
Energy 297kcal/1241kJ;
Protein 12g; Carbohydrate 49g,
of which sugars 11g; Fat 7g, of
which saturates 2g; Cholesterol
19mg; Calcium 58mg; Fibre 1g;
Sodium 341mg

Soups, Snacks & Appetizers

SERVES 4

175g/6oz/1 cup Thai jasmine
   rice
350ml/12fl oz/1½ cups water
oil, for deep-frying and
   greasing

For the spicy dipping sauce
6–8 dried chillies
2.5ml/½ tsp salt
4 coriander (cilantro) roots
10 white peppercorns
250ml/8fl oz/1 cup coconut milk
5ml/1 tsp shrimp paste
115g/4oz minced (ground) pork
55g/2oz tomatoes, chopped
15ml/1 tbsp Thai fish sauce
15ml/1 tbsp palm sugar
   (jaggery) or light muscovado
   (brown) sugar
30ml/2 tbsp tamarind juice
   (tamarind paste mixed with
   warm water)
30ml/2 tbsp coarsely chopped
   roasted peanuts

Start making the rice cakes. Wash the rice in several changes of water. Put it in a pan, add the water and cover tightly. Bring to the boil, reduce the heat and simmer gently for 15 minutes. Preheat the oven to the lowest setting.

Remove the lid and fluff up the rice. Spoon it on to a greased baking sheet and press it down with the back of a spoon. Leave in the oven to dry out overnight.

The next day, make the sauce. Snap off the stems of the chillies, shake out the seeds and soak the chillies in warm water for 20 minutes. Drain and crush in a mortar with the salt. Add the coriander roots and peppercorns and pound to a paste.

Pour the coconut milk into a large pan and bring to the boil. When it begins to separate, stir in the chilli paste. Cook for 2–3 minutes then stir in the shrimp paste.

Add the pork, breaking up any lumps. Cook for 5–10 minutes, then stir in the tomatoes, fish sauce, sugar and tamarind juice. Simmer, stirring occasionally, until the sauce thickens, then stir in the chopped peanuts. Remove from the heat.

Break the rice into pieces. Heat the oil in a wok and deep-fry, in batches, for about 1 minute, until they puff up but are not browned. Remove, drain and serve with the dipping sauce.

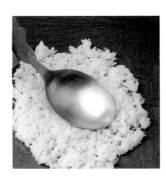
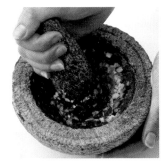

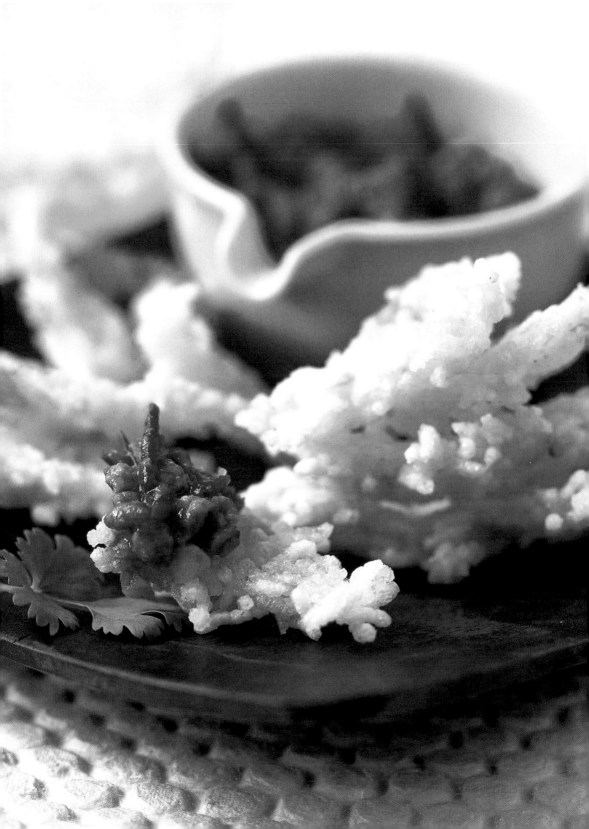

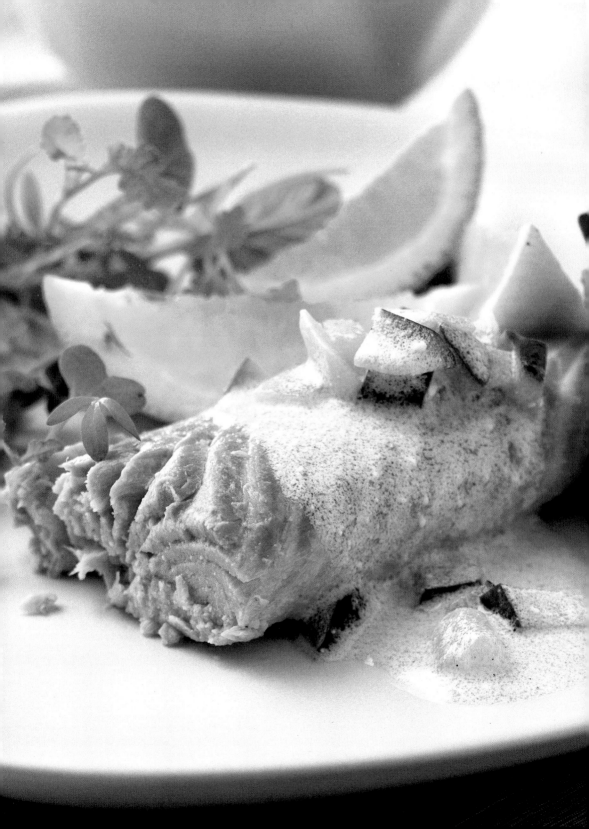

FISH & SHELLFISH

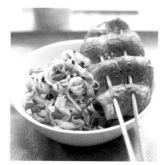
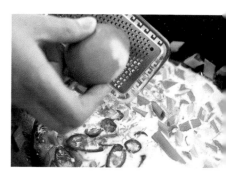

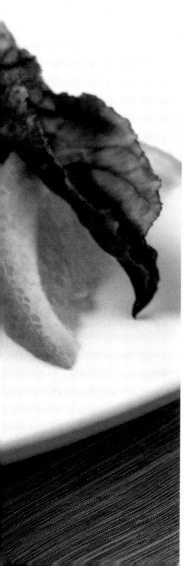

Fish is FODMAP-friendly, and should remain very much part of your healthy, balanced diet. This chapter includes some tasty recipes for oily fish, which should be eaten regularly for essential Omega 3 heart-healthy fats.

SEA BASS WITH FETA AND HERBS

A sustaining mixture of oats, feta cheese, egg and herbs is used to stuff these omega-3-rich sea bass. If sea bass isn't available you can also use trout or red snapper for this recipe. Be careful not to overcook the fish.

FODMAP TYPE: Lactose
NUTRITIONAL CONTENT:
Energy 302kcal/1262kJ;
Protein 31g; Carbohydrate 1g,
of which sugars 1g; Fat 19g, of
which saturates 11g; Cholesterol
150mg; Calcium 294mg; Fibre
Trace; Sodium 596mg

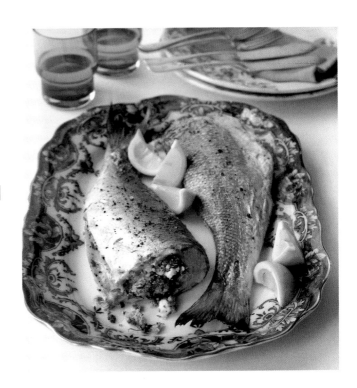

SERVES 4

4 medium sea bass, cleaned, gutted, head removed
juice of 1 lemon
115g/4oz feta cheese
75g/3oz/⅔ cup oats
1 egg white
6 tarragon sprigs, leaves finely chopped
6 thyme sprigs, leaves chopped
8 parsley sprigs, leaves finely chopped
50g/2oz/4 tbsp butter, melted
salt and ground black pepper
lemon wedges, to serve

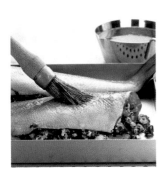

Preheat the oven to 180°C/350°F/Gas 4. Rinse the fish and pat dry with kitchen paper. Rub with the lemon juice and season with salt and pepper.

Crumble the feta cheese into a bowl, and add the oats, egg white and herbs. Mix well to combine.

Spoon some of the filling into the cavity of each fish, then secure with cocktail sticks (toothpicks) and place on a greased baking sheet.

Brush the fish with the melted butter, season with a little salt and pepper and bake for 45–50 minutes, or until cooked through. Serve with lemon wedges.

BAKED BREAM

This is a simple recipe with stunning results that combines fresh fish, potato and herbs. Many hard cheeses, including Italian Pecorino, are low in lactose so shouldn't contribute to any IBS symptoms.

Preheat the oven to 200°C/400°F/Gas 6. Rinse the fish thoroughly and pat it dry. Use half of the oil to coat the fish, inside and out. Season with salt and pepper and tuck half the parsley into the cavity.

Put the potatoes into a baking dish that is large enough to hold the fish. Add the rest of the oil with the remaining parsley. Mix well. Spread the potatoes evenly in the dish, season them with salt and pepper, then sprinkle with the cheese.

Lay the fish on top of the potatoes. Bake for about 40 minutes or until the potatoes are tender and the fish is cooked through, basting occasionally with a little olive oil. Serve the fish and potatoes immediately, straight from the baking dish.

FODMAP TYPE: Lactose
NUTRITIONAL CONTENT:
Energy 682kcal/2851kJ;
Protein 53g; Carbohydrate 22g, of which sugars 1g; Fat 43g, of which saturates 8g; Cholesterol 112mg; Calcium 308mg; Fibre 2g; Sodium 425mg

SERVES 4

1 gilthead bream, about 1kg/2¼lb weight, cleaned and scaled
150ml/¼ pint/⅔ cup extra virgin olive oil, plus extra for basting
a handful of fresh flat leaf parsley, chopped
500g/1¼lb potatoes, peeled and sliced
75g/3oz Pecorino cheese, grated
sea salt and ground black pepper

Fish & Shellfish

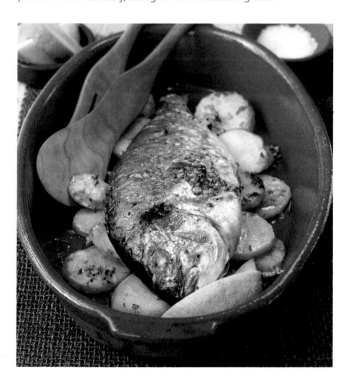

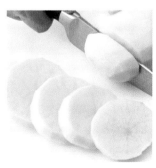

TUNA WITH POLENTA

Polenta is a wheat-free classic Italian staple and is very simple to prepare. Tomato purée usually contains just concentrated tomatoes, but it's worth checking the ingredients to make sure it is onion- and garlic-free.

FODMAP TYPE: Nil
NUTRITIONAL CONTENT:
Energy 680kcal/2842kJ;
Protein 29g; Carbohydrate 79g,
of which sugars 2g; Fat 29g, of
which saturates 4g; Cholesterol
42mg; Calcium 54mg; Fibre 8g;
Sodium 608mg

SERVES 2

200g/7oz/¾ cup polenta
150g/5oz canned tuna, flaked
4 anchovy fillets, rinsed
60ml/4 tbsp virgin olive oil
a small handful of fresh flat
    leaf parsley leaves, chopped
a small handful of celery leaves,
    chopped
30ml/2 tbsp tomato purée
    (paste) diluted in 30ml/2 tbsp
    hot water or fish stock
sea salt and ground black
    pepper

First make the polenta. Bring 1.75 litres/3 pints/7½ cups water in a pan to the boil and add a large pinch of salt, then slowly trickle the polenta flour into the water, whisking constantly.

Over a medium-low heat, stir the polenta constantly for 45 minutes, or until it comes away from the sides of the pan.

Finely chop the tuna with the anchovies. Put the oil in a pan and fry the parsley, celery leaves and fish together for 5 minutes, then stir in the diluted tomato purée. Season with pepper and simmer the sauce for about 30 minutes.

To serve pour the soft polenta into individual bowls and add the fish topping to each.

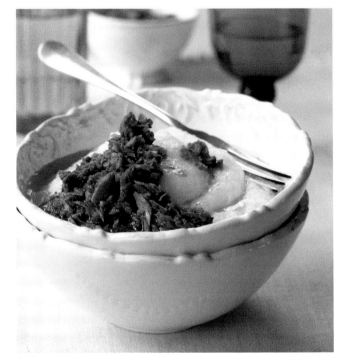

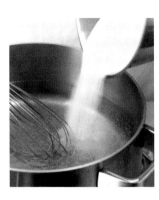

ROASTED FISH WITH CHILLIES AND WALNUTS

Although red snapper is usually used in this recipe, you can use any firm white-fleshed fish for this fiery, Lebanese dish. Pomegranate seeds and molasses are fine in limited amounts, adding a distinct, combination of sweet and sour.

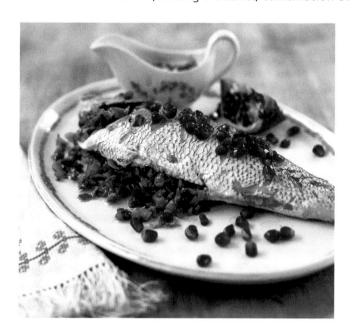

FODMAP TYPE: Fructans
NUTRITIONAL CONTENT:
Energy 728kcal/3043kJ;
Protein 97g; Carbohydrate 7g,
of which sugars 6g; Fat 35g, of
which saturates 4g; Cholesterol
166mg; Calcium 347mg; Fibre
2g; Sodium 360mg

SERVES 4

2 x 900g/2lb firm-fleshed fish,
   gutted and cleaned
60ml/4 tbsp olive oil
1 green (bell) pepper, finely
   chopped
1–2 red chillies, seeded and
   very finely chopped
115g/4oz walnuts, chopped
15–30ml/1–2 tbsp pomegranate
   molasses
small bunch of fresh coriander
   (cilantro), finely chopped
small bunch of flat leaf parsley,
   finely chopped
sea salt and black pepper

For the sauce
60ml/4 tbsp tahini
juice of 1 lemon
juice of 1 orange
15ml/1 tbsp olive oil
1–2 red chillies, finely chopped
sea salt and black pepper
seeds of ½ pomegranate,
   to garnish

Preheat the oven to 200°C/400°F/Gas 6.Cut three slits on each side of the fish. Rub the cavity with salt and pepper, cover the fish and chill for 30 minutes.

Heat 30ml/2 tbsp olive oil in a heavy pan and fry the chopped pepper and chillies until for 3–4 minutes. Stir in the walnuts and pomegranate molasses and add the coriander and parsley. Season to taste and leave the filling to cool.

Fill the fish with the stuffing and secure the opening with a wooden skewer. Place the fish in an oiled baking dish and pour over the remaining oil. Bake for about 30 minutes.

To make the sauce, beat the tahini with the lemon and orange juice until smooth and creamy. Heat the oil in a small pan and stir in the chillies, then add the tahini mixture and heat through. Garnish the cooked fish with the pomegranate seeds and a drizzle of sauce and serve with the rest of the sauce.

FISH GRATIN

Serve this hearty winter supper dish either on its own, or with wheat-free bread or potato. Make sure you use suitable (onion- and garlic-free) fish stock, or use water and add additional herbs and seasoning to taste.

FODMAP TYPE: Lactose
NUTRITIONAL CONTENT:
Energy 595kcal/2487kJ;
Protein 38g; Carbohydrate 10g, of which sugars 1g; Fat 42g, of which saturates 23g; Cholesterol 223mg; Calcium 321mg; Fibre 1g; Sodium 727mg

Fish & Shellfish

SERVES 4

l litre/1¾ pints/4 cups onion-free fish stock
400g/14oz firm fish fillets, such as monkfish, salmon, turbot or cod, cut into cubes
200g/7oz cooked prawns (shrimps) or/and shelled cooked mussels, or peeled uncooked scampi (extra large shrimp)
40g/1½oz/⅓ cup cornflour (cornstarch)
100g/3½oz/scant ½ cup butter
100ml/3½fl oz/scant ½ cup dry white wine or dry vermouth
100ml/3½fl oz/scant ½ cup double (heavy) cream
115g/4oz/1 cup grated mature (sharp) Cheddar cheese
45ml/3 tbsp chopped fresh parsley
salt and ground white pepper

Preheat the oven to 200°C/400°F/Gas 6. Grease a 1.2 litre/2 pint/5 cup baking dish.

Bring the fish stock to the boil in a large pan. Add the fish cubes, reduce the heat and poach for 2 minutes. If using scampi, poach them for 1 minute, until barely pink.

As soon as the fish pieces are cooked, lift them out with a slotted spoon and layer in the dish. Season and cover to keep warm. Pour the fish stock into a measuring jug (cup).

Place the cornflour in a small bowl, and blend with 30ml/2 tbsp of the reserved fish stock to a smooth paste. Add the remaining stock and transfer to a pan, heat until thickened, stirring all the time. Add the butter, wine or vermouth, cream, and seasoning, and stir until smooth.

Remove from the heat and add most of the grated cheese, reserving about 45ml/3 tbsp for the topping. Stir in the grey shrimps and/or mussels, with 15ml/1 tbsp of the parsley, and spoon over the fish. Sprinkle with the reserved cheese.

Bake for 10–15 minutes, until the cheese turns golden. Sprinkle with the remaining parsley and serve immediately.

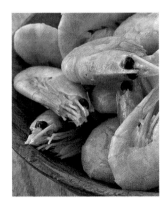
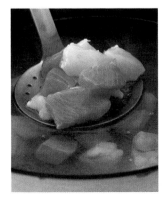

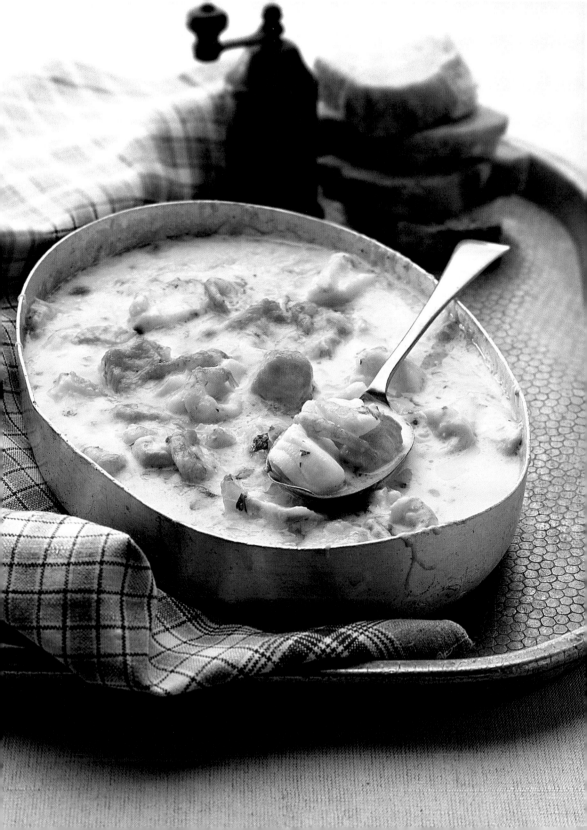

SPAGHETTI WITH TUNA AND ANCHOVIES

There is an increasing selection of wheat-free pastas available, which means you can safely eat many of your favourite Italian-style recipes on the low-FODMAP diet. This dish also contains mozzarella, which is low in lactose.

FODMAP TYPE: Lactose
NUTRITIONAL CONTENT:
Energy 551kcal/2303kJ;
Protein 26g; Carbohydrate 72g,
of which sugars 9g Fat 19g, of
which saturates 7g; Cholesterol
52mg; Calcium 174mg; Fibre 3g;
Sodium 1103mg

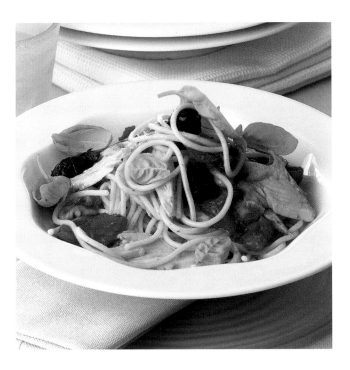

Fish & Shellfish

SERVES 4

300g/11oz dried gluten-free
    spaghetti
30ml/2 tbsp olive oil
6 ripe Italian plum tomatoes,
    chopped
5ml/1 tsp sugar
50g/2oz anchovies in olive oil,
    drained
about 60ml/4 tbsp dry white
    wine
200g/7oz can tuna in olive oil,
    drained
50g/2oz/½ cup pitted black
    olives, quartered lengthways
125g/4½oz mozzarella cheese,
    drained and diced
salt and ground black pepper
basil leaves, to serve

VARIATION Use the same
quantities of prawns (shrimp)
and capers instead of tuna
and anchovies, if you wish.

Cook the pasta according to the instructions on the packet. Meanwhile, heat the oil in a medium pan.

Add the tomatoes, sugar and pepper to taste to the pan, and toss over a medium heat for a few minutes until the tomatoes soften and the juices run.

Snip a few anchovies at a time into the pan with kitchen scissors and add the wine, tuna and olives. Stir once or twice until they are just evenly mixed into the sauce. Add the mozzarella and heat through without stirring, until the cheese starts to melt. Taste and add salt if necessary.

Drain the pasta and transfer it into a warmed bowl. Pour the sauce over, toss gently, sprinkle with basil leaves and serve.

SALMON WITH CUCUMBER SAUCE

Sautéed cucumber laced with dill and sour cream is an unusual accompaniment to salmon, served either warm, or cooled as a light lunch. Moderate dashes of wine and sour cream add decadence without overdoing the FODMAPs.

Season the salmon and brush inside and out with melted butter. Place the herb sprigs and lemon in the cavity. Preheat the oven to 220°C/425°F/Gas 7.

Wrap the salmon in foil, folding the edges together securely, and bake for 15 minutes. Remove the fish from the oven but leave in the foil for 1 hour.

Meanwhile, halve the cucumber lengthways, scoop out the seeds, then dice the flesh. Place the cucumber in a colander, toss lightly with salt and leave for about 30 minutes to drain. Rinse well, drain again and pat dry.

Heat the butter in a small pan, add the cucumber and cook for 2 minutes until translucent. Add the wine and boil briskly until the cucumber is dry. Stir in the dill and sour cream and season to taste. Serve the salmon with the cucumber sauce, orange slices and salad leaves.

FODMAP TYPE: Lactose
NUTRITIONAL CONTENT:
Energy 649kcal/2713kJ;
Protein 62g; Carbohydrate 2g, of which sugars 2g; Fat 42g, of which saturates 12g; Cholesterol 175mg; Calcium 98mg; Fibre 1g; Sodium 182mg

SERVES 6

1.8kg/4lb salmon, cleaned and scaled
melted butter, for brushing
3 fresh parsley or thyme sprigs
½ lemon, halved
orange slices and salad leaves, to serve

For the cucumber sauce
1 large cucumber, peeled
25g/1oz/2 tbsp butter
120ml/4fl oz/½ cup dry white wine
45ml/3 tbsp finely chopped fresh dill
60ml/4 tbsp sour cream
salt and ground black pepper

COOK'S TIP The cucumber needs to be de-seeded otherwise they seeds will break away during cooking and spoil the texture of the sauce.

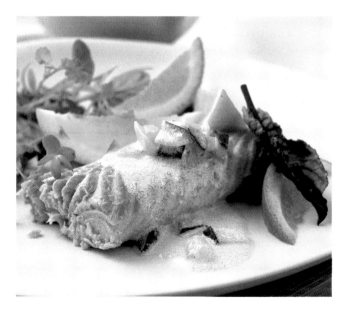

TERIYAKI SALMON

Mirin is a sweetened version of Japanese rice wine, which combined with soy sauce forms an intensely-flavoured Teryaki glaze. Sake is usually fructose-free, but check the ingredients of the mirin, as some brands do include fructose.

FODMAP TYPE: Nil
NUTRITIONAL CONTENT:
Energy 402kcal/1680kJ;
Protein 31g Carbohydrate 17g, of which sugars 16g; Fat 23g, of which saturates 4g; Cholesterol 75mg; Calcium 39mg; Fibre 0g; Sodium 1403mg

SERVES 4

75ml/5 tbsp soy sauce
75ml/5 tbsp mirin
75ml/5 tbsp sake
15ml/1 tbsp sugar
4 salmon fillets, about 150g/5oz each
5cm/2in piece of fresh root ginger, peeled and cut into matchsticks
sunflower oil, for frying
steamed rice, to serve

In a bowl, mix the soy sauce, mirin, sake and sugar together. Place the salmon fillets in the bowl and marinade for up to 2 hours in the refrigerator.

Heat a good amount of sunflower oil in a small pan and add the ginger. Fry for 1–2 minutes, until golden and crisp. Remove with a slotted spoon and drain on kitchen paper.

Heat the grill (broiler) until hot. Remove the salmon from the marinade and place in a roasting pan, skin side down, and drizzle a little marinade over the top.

Grill (broil) for 2–3 minutes, then turn over and cook for a further 1–2 minutes. Turn over again so skin side is down, drizzle a little more marinade over the top and grill for a further 1–2 minutes until cooked through and crispy.

Remove from the pan and divide among four serving plates. Top the salmon fillets with the crispy fried ginger.

Pour the remaining marinade into a small pan and bring to the boil, simmer for 1–2 minutes, then drizzle over the salmon and serve with steamed rice.

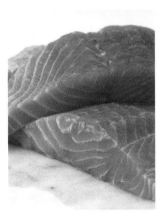
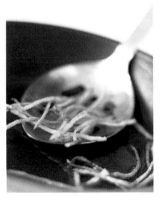

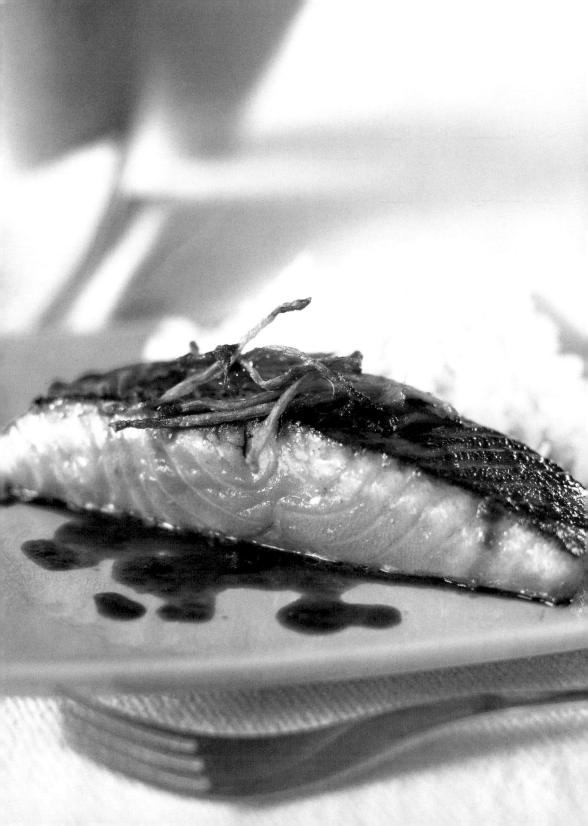

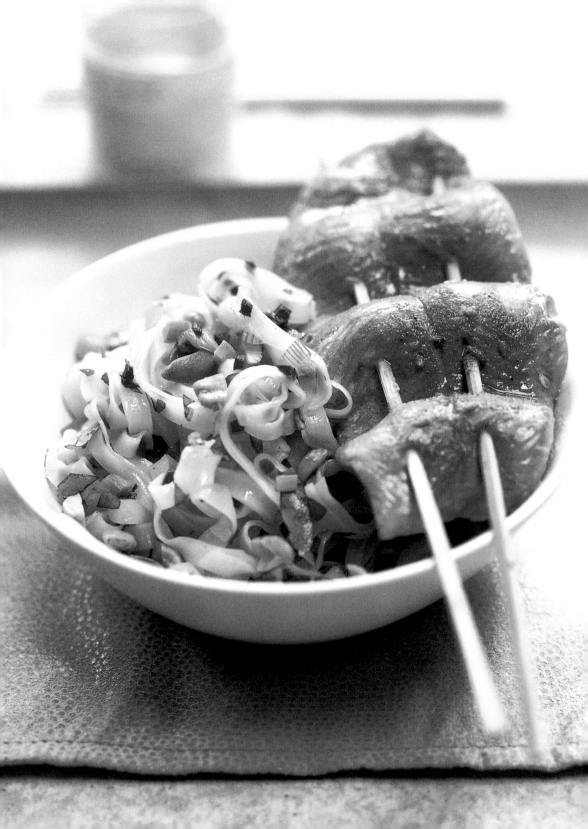

STEAMED FISH SKEWERS ON HERBED RICE NOODLES

Avoiding onion and garlic is tricky on a low-FODMAP diet, but fortunately a range of herbs and spices are suitable, and are used in this curried fish recipe. Use curry powder, not paste, which often contains garlic.

Trim each fillet and place in a large bowl. Mix together the turmeric, curry powder, lemon juice and oil and pour over the fish. Season with salt and black pepper and toss to mix well.

Place the rice noodles in a bowl and pour over enough boiling water to cover. Leave to soak for 3–4 minutes and then drain. Refresh in cold water, drain and set aside.

Thread 2 bamboo skewers through each trout fillet and arrange in two tiers of a steamer lined with baking parchment.

Cover the steamer and place over a wok of simmering water (making sure the water doesn't touch the steamer). Steam the fish skewers for 5–6 minutes, or until the fish is just cooked through and flakes easily.

Meanwhile, in a clean wok heat the oil. Add the chilli, spring onions and drained noodles and stir-fry for about 2 minutes. Stir in the chopped herbs. Season with salt and ground black pepper and divide among four bowls or plates.

Top each bowl of noodles with a steamed fish skewer and scatter over the chilli-roasted peanuts. Garnish with chopped mint and serve immediately.

FODMAP TYPE: Nil
NUTRITIONAL CONTENT:
Energy 582kcal/2433kJ;
Protein 37g; Carbohydrate 65g,
of which sugars 2g; Fat 18g, of
which saturates 2g; Cholesterol
0mg; Calcium 144mg; Fibre 1g;
Sodium 157mg

SERVES 4

4 trout fillets, skinned
2.5ml/½ tsp turmeric
15ml/1 tbsp mild curry powder
juice of 2 lemons
15ml/1 tbsp sunflower oil
salt and ground black pepper
45ml/3 tbsp chilli-roasted
    peanuts, roughly chopped
chopped fresh mint, to garnish

For the noodles
300g/11oz rice noodles
15ml/1 tbsp sunflower oil
1 red chilli, seeded and finely
    sliced
4 spring onions (scallions),
    green parts only, cut into
    thin rounds
60ml/4 tbsp roughly chopped
    fresh mint
60ml/4 tbsp roughly chopped
    fresh sweet basil

Fish & Shellfish

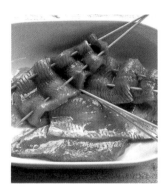
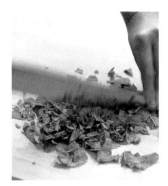

SPICED HALIBUT CURRY

Most Indian spices are FODMAP-free, but some IBS sufferers might find that richly spiced foods do affect them. Reduce or omit the chilli powder in this recipe if you want a milder flavour, or add spring onion greens to sharpen it up a bit.

Fish & Shellfish

FODMAP TYPE: Lactose
NUTRITIONAL CONTENT:
Energy 321kcal/1342kJ;
Protein 43g; Carbohydrate 4g,
of which sugars 3g; Fat 18g, of
which saturates 2g; Cholesterol
66mg; Calcium 156mg; Fibre 1g;
Sodium 649mg

SERVES 4

60ml/4 tbsp lemon juice
60ml/4 tbsp rice wine vinegar
30ml/2 tbsp cumin seeds
5ml/1 tsp turmeric
5ml/1 tsp chilli powder
5ml/1 tsp salt
750g/1lb 11oz thick halibut
    fillets, skinned and cubed
60ml/4 tbsp sunflower oil
30ml/2 tbsp finely grated fresh
    root ginger
10ml/2 tsp black mustard seeds
pinch of asafoetida
200g/7oz canned chopped
    tomatoes
5ml/1 tsp sugar
chopped coriander (cilantro)
    and sliced green chilli, to
    garnish
crème fraîche (optional)
basmati rice, to serve

Mix together the lemon juice, vinegar, cumin, turmeric, chilli powder and salt in a shallow glass bowl. Add the cubed fish and turn to coat evenly. Cover and put in the refrigerator to marinate for 25–30 minutes.

Meanwhile, heat a wok over a high heat and add the oil. When hot, add the ginger, mustard seeds and asafoetida. Reduce the heat to low and cook, stirring, for a few seconds.

Add the tomatoes and sugar to the wok, bring to a boil, reduce the heat, cover and cook gently for 10–12 minutes, stirring occasionally.

Add the fish and its marinade to the wok, stir gently to mix, then cover and simmer gently for 12–15 minutes, or until the fish is just cooked through and flakes easily with a fork.

Serve the curry ladled into shallow bowls with basmati rice. Garnish with fresh coriander and green chillies, and drizzle over some crème fraîche if liked.

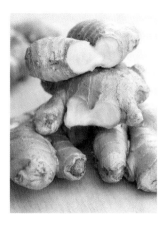
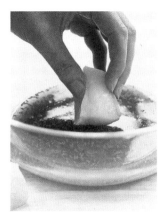

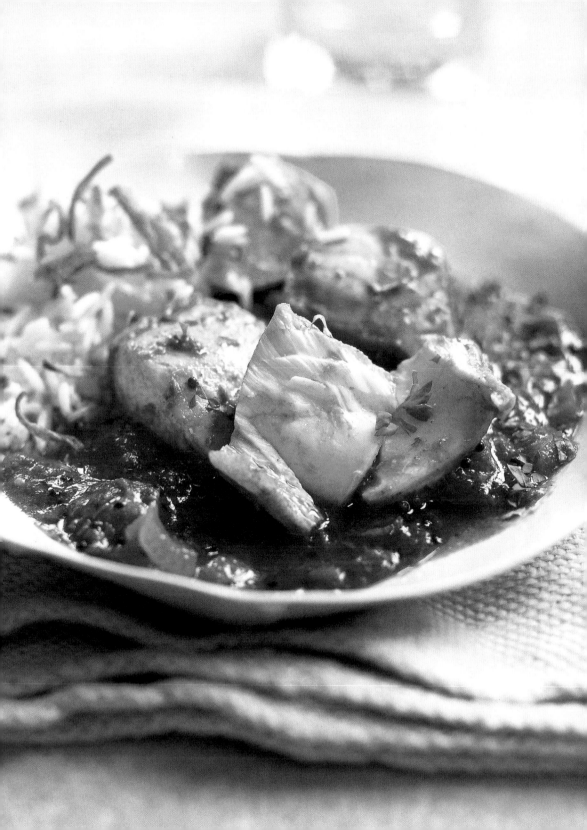

SEAFOOD RICE

This recipe is very similar to Spanish paella and reminiscent of long lunches in the sun. All fish and seafood is FODMAP-free, and if you make use of frozen, bagged mixes this can make a great store cupboard standby.

FODMAP TYPE: Nil
NUTRITIONAL CONTENT:
Energy 555kcal/2320kJ;
Protein 42g; Carbohydrate 61g,
of which sugars 2g; Fat 14g, of
which saturates 4g; Cholesterol
185mg; Calcium 162mg; Fibre
2g; Sodium 642mg

SERVES 4

50ml/2fl oz/¼ cup olive oil
1 green (bell) pepper, seeded
    and chopped
1 tomato, peeled and chopped
1 litre/1¾ pints/4 cups fish stock
200g/7oz live clams, scrubbed
200g/7oz live cockles, scrubbed
200g/7oz live mussels, scrubbed
    and beards removed
300g/11oz/1½ cups risotto rice
400g/14oz cooked peeled
    prawns (shrimp)
30ml/2 tbsp chopped fresh
    coriander (cilantro)

Heat the olive oil in a large pan. Add the green pepper and cook over a low heat, stirring occasionally, for 5 minutes, until softened. Add the tomato and the stock and bring to the boil.

Open the clams, cockles and mussels. The easiest way do this is by steaming them briefly in a little water and removing them from their shells when opened. Discard any that do not open. Reserve the shellfish meat, keeping the shells to one side.

Add the rice to the pan, bring back to the boil and cook for about 12 minutes, until tender. The mixture should be moist; if necessary, add more stock. Add all the seafood and the coriander to the pan, heat through briefly and serve, decorated with the seafood shells.

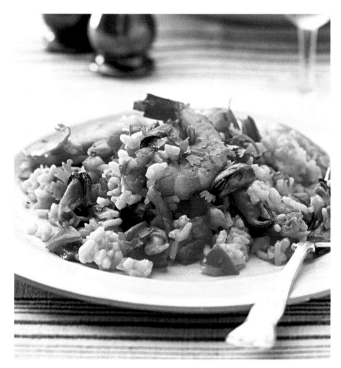

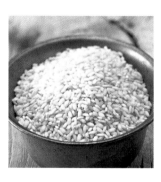

TANGY PRAWN KEBABS

Sweet and sour pomegranate molasses (made from the seeds and sugar) gives these kebabs a delicious mellow sweetness, and is fine in controlled quantities. Grill on the barbecue if possible, and serve with rice or new potatoes.

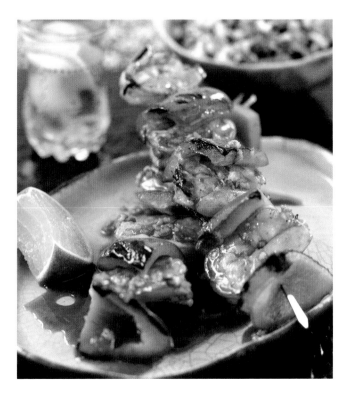

FODMAP TYPE: Fructans
NUTRITIONAL CONTENT:
Energy 168kcal/702kJ;
Protein 23g; Carbohydrate 6g, of which sugars 5g; Fat 5g, of which saturates 1g; Cholesterol 160mg; Calcium 112mg; Fibre 0g; Sodium 197mg

SERVES 4

Fish & Shellfish

15ml/1 tbsp pomegranate molasses
15ml/1 tbsp olive oil
juice of 1 lemon
10ml/2 tsp sugar
16 large raw prawns (shrimp), shelled and deveined
2 green (bell) peppers, cut into bitesize chunks
sea salt
lime wedges, to serve

In a large bowl, mix together the pomegranate molasses, olive oil, lemon juice and sugar. Season the mixture with salt.

Add the prawns to the mixture, and toss gently, making sure they are all well coated with the marinade. Cover the dish and marinate in the refrigerator for 1–2 hours.

Prepare the barbecue, if using, or preheat a griddle or grill (broiler). Thread the marinated prawns on to four skewers, alternately with the pepper pieces.

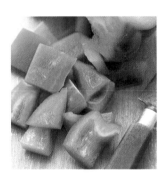

Grill the kebabs for 2–3 minutes on each side, basting with any leftover marinade. Serve immediately with wedges of lime.

TIGER PRAWNS WITH CUCUMBER AND DILL

Cucumber, courgette and marrow, from the cucurbit family, are all FODMAP-free, making them very handy bases for all sorts of dishes. Here, cucumber is teamed up with delicate dill, and can be served with steamed rice, quinoa or buckwheat.

FODMAP TYPE: Nil
NUTRITIONAL CONTENT:
Energy 229kcal/957kJ;
Protein 27g; Carbohydrate 2g,
of which sugars 2g; Fat 11g, of
which saturates 5g; Cholesterol
216mg; Calcium 148mg; Fibre
1g; Sodium 582mg

Fish & Shellfish

SERVES 4

500g/1¼lb raw tiger prawns
   (jumbo shrimp), peeled and
   deveined but with tail on
500g/1¼lb cucumber
30ml/2 tbsp butter
15ml/1 tbsp olive oil
45ml/3 tbsp chopped fresh dill
juice of 1 lemon
salt and ground black pepper
steamed rice or quinoa,
   to serve

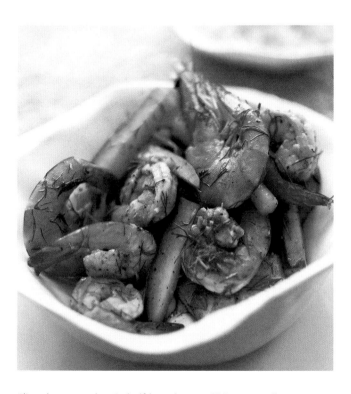

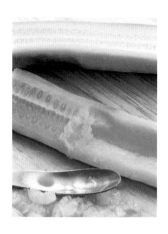

Slice the cucumber in half lengthways. Using a small teaspoon, gently scoop out all the seeds and discard. Cut the cucumber into 4 x 1cm/1½ x ½in sticks.

Heat a wok over a high heat, then add the butter and oil. When the butter has melted, add the cucumber and stir-fry over a high heat for 2–3 minutes.

Add the prepared prawns to the wok and continue to stir-fry over a high heat for 3–4 minutes, or until the prawns turn pink and are just cooked through, then remove from the heat.

Add the dill and lemon juice to the wok and toss to combine. Season and serve immediately with steamed rice or quinoa.

SCALLOPS WITH BACON AND SAGE

Like thyme and rosemary, sage is ideal for adding precious flavour to low-FODMAP cooking. A dash of wine or cider also intensifies the flavour of this dish which is great as a main course for two, served with rice, or an appetizer for four.

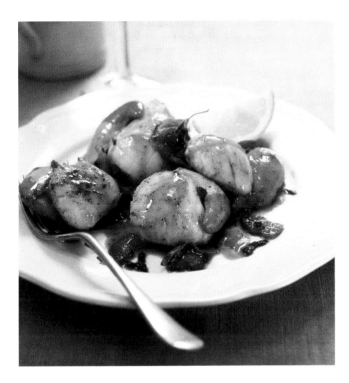

FODMAP TYPE: Nil
NUTRITIONAL CONTENT:
Energy 433kcal/1810kJ;
Protein 53g; Carbohydrate 7g,
of which sugars Trace; Fat 17g, of
which saturates 5g; Cholesterol
119mg; Calcium 65mg; Fibre 0g;
Sodium 865mg

SERVES 2

15ml/1 tbsp olive oil
4 streaky (fatty) bacon rashers
   (strips), cut into 2.5cm/
   1in pieces
2–3 fresh sage leaves, chopped
small piece of butter
8 large or 16 small scallops
15ml/1 tbsp fresh lemon juice
100ml/3¾fl oz dry (hard) cider
   or dry white wine
lemon wedges, to serve

Heat the oil in a frying pan. Add the bacon and sage and cook, stirring occasionally, until the bacon is golden brown. Lift out and keep warm.

Add the butter to the pan and when hot add the scallops. Cook quickly for about 1 minute on each side until browned. Lift out and keep warm.

Add the lemon juice and cider or wine to the pan and, scraping up any sediment remaining in the pan, bring just to the boil.

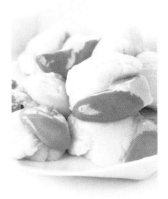

Continue bubbling gently until the mixture has reduced to just a few tablespoons of syrupy sauce. Serve the scallops and bacon with the sauce drizzled over and lemon wedges.

THAI-STYLE STEAMED MUSSELS

This dish features classic ingredients of Thai cooking, including low-FODMAP chillies, limes and coconut milk, making a hot and aromatic lunch or supper dish. Use other seafood such as clams or squid if you prefer.

FODMAP TYPE: Sorbitol
NUTRITIONAL CONTENT:
Energy 169kcal/706kJ;
Protein 22g; Carbohydrate 8g,
of which sugars 8g; Fat 6g, of
which saturates 1g; Cholesterol
47mg; Calcium 278mg; Fibre
Trace; Sodium 1166mg

SERVES 4

1.6kg/3½lb live mussels
15ml/1 tbsp sunflower oil
15ml/1 tbsp finely chopped
    fresh root ginger
2 large red chillies, seeded and
    finely sliced
6 spring onions (scallions),
    green parts only, finely
    chopped
400ml/14fl oz/1⅔ cups coconut
    milk
45ml/3 tbsp light soy sauce
finely grated zest and juice of
    2 limes
5ml/1 tsp caster (superfine)
    sugar
a large handful of fresh
    chopped coriander (cilantro)
salt and ground black pepper

Scrub the mussels in clean running water, removing any beards, and throwing away any mussels that are open and do not close when lightly tapped.

Heat the wok over a high heat and then add the oil. Stir in the chopped ginger, chillies and spring onion greens and cook, stirring continuously for 30 seconds.

Pour the coconut milk into the wok and add the soy sauce, lime and sugar, stirring stir to mix.

Bring the spiced coconut milk to the boil, then add the mussels. Return to the boil, cover and cook briskly for 5–6 minutes, or until all the mussels have opened. Discard any unopened mussels.

Remove the wok from the heat and stir in the chopped coriander. Season the mussels well with salt and pepper. Ladle into warmed bowls and serve immediately.

COOK'S TIP Make use of pre-chopped, chilled, Thai ingredients such as chilli paste, chopped ginger and frozen coriander leaves for speedier preparation.

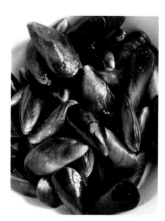
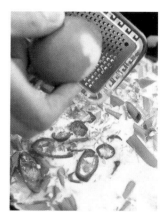

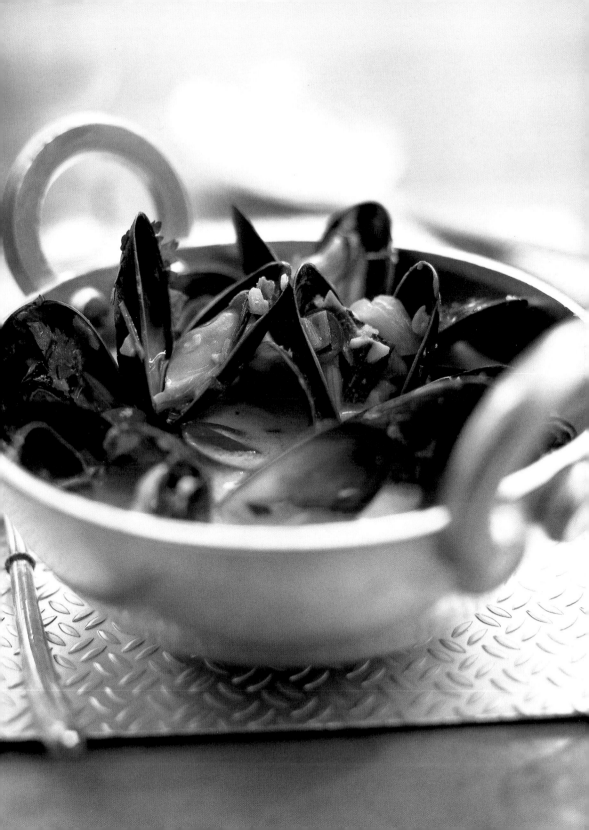

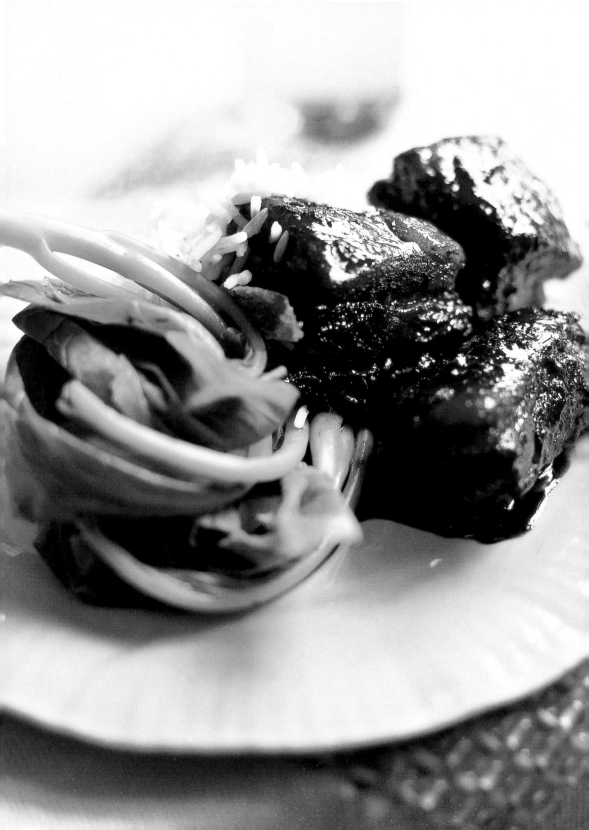

MEAT

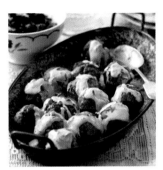 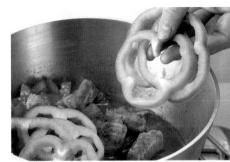

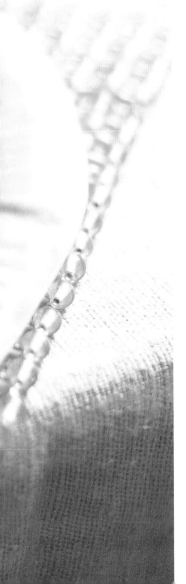

Cooking without onion and garlic needn't be a barrier to delicious, memorable meals. This chapter makes use of alternatives such as asafoetida powder, which is used in Asian cooking and gives an onion-like flavour on heating. Garlic-infused oil, spices and herbs are also used to great effect.

ROAST LIME CHICKEN WITH SWEET POTATOES

This recipe is a tasty twist on simple roast chicken, using fresh and dried turmeric, lime juice and soy sauce. Accompanying sweet potato contains some of the FODMAP, polyol, but the controlled portions used here are fine.

FODMAP TYPE: (Polyol) Mannitol
NUTRITIONAL CONTENT:
Energy 530kcal/2215kJ;
Protein 52g; Carbohydrate 11g,
of which sugars 4.4g; Fat 32g, of
which saturates 9g; Cholesterol
221mg; Calcium 43mg; Fibre 2g;
Sodium 902mg

Meat

SERVES 4

small bunch coriander
   (cilantro), with roots,
   coarsely chopped
5ml/1 tsp ground turmeric
5cm/2in piece fresh turmeric
1 roasting chicken, about
   1.5kg/3¼lb in weight
1 lime, cut in half
1 medium sweet potato, and
   3 large parsnips, peeled
   and cut into thick wedges
300ml/½ pint/1¼ cups low-
   FODMAP chicken stock
30ml/2 tbsp soy sauce
salt and ground black pepper

VARIATION Mix and match
the proportion of sweet
potato and parsnip, or use
ordinary potatoes and carrots
instead, if you prefer.

Preheat the oven to 190°C/375°F/Gas 5. Calculate the cooking time for the chicken, allowing 20 minutes per 500g/1¼lb, plus 20 minutes. With a mortar and pestle or food processor, grind the coriander, 10ml/2 tsp salt and turmeric to a paste.

Place the chicken in a roasting pan and smear it with the paste. Squeeze the lime juice over and place the lime halves in the cavity. Cover with foil and roast in the oven.

Meanwhile, bring a pan of water to the boil and par-boil the sweet potato and parsnips for 10–15 minutes, until just tender. Drain well and place them around the chicken in the roasting pan. Baste with the cooking juices and sprinkle with salt and pepper. Replace the foil and return the chicken to the oven.

About 20 minutes before the end of cooking, remove the foil and baste the chicken. Turn the sweet potato and parsnips over.

At the end of the calculated roasting time, check that the chicken is cooked. Lift it out of the roasting pan, tip it so that all the juices collected in the cavity drain into the pan, then place the bird on a carving board.

Cover the chicken with tented foil and leave it to rest before carving. Transfer the vegetables to a serving dish and keep them hot in the oven while you make the gravy.

Pour away the oil from the roasting pan but keep the juices. Place the roasting pan on top of the stove and heat until the juices are bubbling. Pour in the stock.

Bring the mixture to the boil, stirring with a wooden spoon and scraping the base of the pan to incorporate the residue.

Stir in the soy sauce and check the seasoning before straining the gravy into a jug or pitcher. Serve it with the carved meat and the roasted vegetables.

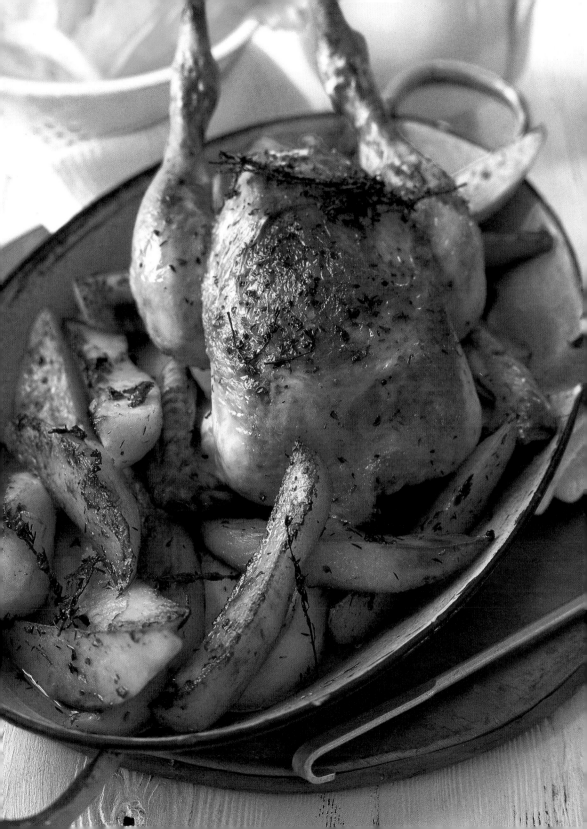

CHICKEN WITH SPICY RED PEPPER SAUCE

This Spanish recipe makes a heart-warming, family supper dish, though you may want to tone down the chilli for younger taste buds. You can't really beat freshly roasted peppers, but use bottled chargrilled peppers in oil if time is tight.

FODMAP TYPE: Nil
NUTRITIONAL CONTENT:
Energy 505kcal/2111kJ;
Protein 37g; Carbohydrate 3g,
of which sugars 2g; Fat 39g, of
which saturates 12g; Cholesterol
155mg; Calcium 76mg; Fibre 4g;
Sodium 1186mg

Remove the seeds and stalks from the peeled peppers and purée the flesh in a food processor.

Rub salt and paprika into the chicken portions. Heat the oil in a large frying pan and fry the chicken over a medium-low heat, turning until golden on all sides. Transfer to a large pan.

Add the chopped tomatoes, puréed peppers, chopped dried chilli or chilli powder to the frying pan. Cook for 2–3 minutes, letting the sauce reduce, then pour over the chicken.

Cover and cook, for 30–45 minutes until the chicken is tender. Check the seasoning, adding salt and pepper if necessary. Garnish with a little parsley and serve with small new potatoes.

Meat

SERVES 4

675g/1½lb red (bell) peppers, grilled (broiled) or roasted in a high oven, to char the skin, and peeled
4 free-range chicken portions
10ml/2 tsp paprika
30ml/2 tbsp olive oil
200g/7oz lardons
115g/4oz canned chopped tomatoes
1 dried guindilla or other hot dried chilli, chopped, or 2.5ml/½ tsp chilli powder, to taste
salt and ground black pepper
chopped fresh parsley, to garnish
small new potatoes, to serve

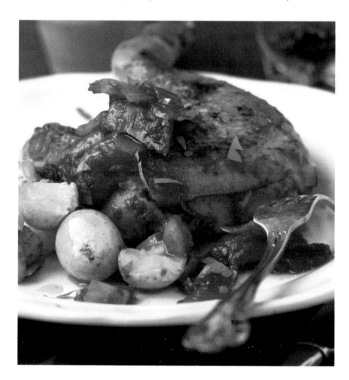

TUSCAN-STYLE CHICKEN

Giblets are full of flavour and useful protein, iron and Vitamin B12, and, like everything else in this recipe are FODMAP-free. Serve with a side of new potatoes and butter-glazed green beans for a complete meal.

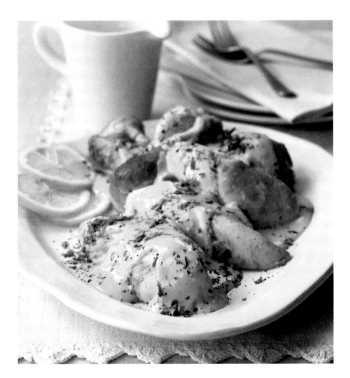

FODMAP TYPE: Nil
NUTRITIONAL CONTENT:
Energy 700kcal/2926kJ;
Protein 60g; Carbohydrate Trace,
of which sugars 0g; Fat 51g, of
which saturates 13g; Cholesterol
348mg; Calcium 32mg; Fibre 0g;
Sodium 498mg

Meat

200g/7oz chicken giblets,
  trimmed
15g/½oz/1 tbsp unsalted butter
90ml/6 tbsp virgin olive oil
1 oven-ready free-range
  chicken, about 3kg/6lb 9oz
onion-free chicken stock,
  as needed
3 eggs, beaten
juice and grated zest of
  ½ large, unwaxed lemon
sea salt
chopped fresh flat leaf parsley
  and lemon slices, to garnish

Put the giblets in a deep pan with a lid over a medium heat and add the butter and olive oil. Cook together for 5 minutes.

Add the chicken to the pan and cook briefly on all sides to seal. Pour in an even mixture of water and chicken stock to come about three-quarters of the way up the pan. Add salt to taste, cover, and simmer gently for about 1½–2 hours until the liquid is almost evaporated. Take the chicken out of the pan, and carve into portions. Remove and discard the giblets.

Whisk together the eggs and the juice and rind of the lemon, and add to the juices left in the pan. Beat until the eggs thicken slightly. Pour the sauce over the chicken portions, sprinkle with parsley and serve garnished with lemon slices.

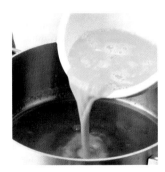

DUCK AND SESAME STIR-FRY

This is a super-speedy supper dish that leaves you wanting for nothing more than a few rice or buckwheat noodles to soak up the tantalizing sauce. Just check that any Thai fish sauce you use is onion- and garlic-free.

FODMAP TYPE: Polyol (Sorbitol)
NUTRITIONAL CONTENT:
Energy 352kcal/1472kJ;
Protein 28g; Carbohydrate 4g,
of which sugars 2g; Fat 24g, of
which saturates 6g; Cholesterol
136mg; Calcium 98mg; Fibre 2g;
Sodium 986mg

Meat

SERVES 2

250g/9oz boneless duck meat
15ml/1 tbsp sesame oil
15ml/1 tbsp vegetable oil
2cm/1in piece fresh ginger,
    grated
2.5ml/½ tsp dried chilli flakes
15ml/1 tbsp Thai fish sauce
15ml/1 tbsp light soy sauce
120ml/4fl oz/½ cup water
115g/4oz broccoli florets
coriander (cilantro) and
    15ml/1tbsp toasted sesame
    seeds, to garnish

Cut the duck meat into bitesize pieces. Heat the oils in a wok or large, heavy frying pan and stir-fry the ginger over a medium heat for a few seconds – do not let it burn.

Add the duck to the pan and stir-fry for a further 2 minutes, until the meat begins to brown.

Stir in the chilli flakes, fish sauce, soy sauce and water. Add the broccoli and continue to stir-fry for about 2 minutes, until the duck is just cooked through.

Serve the duck and broccoli on warmed plates, garnished with coriander and sesame seeds.

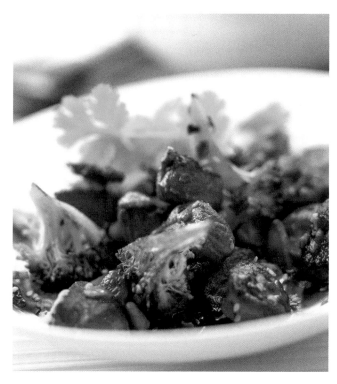

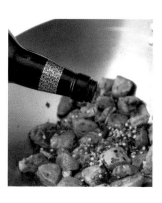

BEEF, CARROT AND SQUASH WITH CHILLI

Butternut squash contains two types of FODMAPs but can be included in small servings. This oriental recipe includes five spice and star anise, which are FODMAP-free and give a lovely warm flavour to the dish.

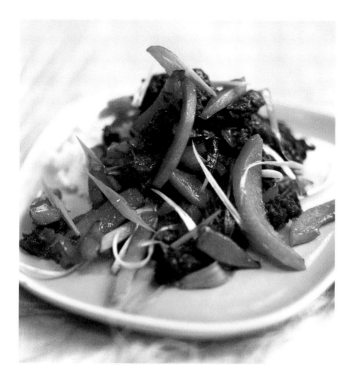

FODMAP: Polyol (Mannitol & GOS)
NUTRITIONAL CONTENT:
Energy 430kcal/1797kJ;
Protein 38g; Carbohydrate 35g,
of which sugars 31g; Fat 17g, of
which saturates 6g; Cholesterol
103mg; Calcium 90mg; Fibre 2g;
Sodium 1481mg

Meat

30ml/2 tbsp sunflower oil
225g/8oz butternut squash,
    peeled, seeded and cut
    into strips
4 medium carrots, peeled and
    cut into strips
675g/1½lb fillet steak (beef
    tenderloin)
60ml/4 tbsp soy sauce
90g/3½oz/½ cup caster
    (superfine) sugar
1 bird's eye chilli, seeded and
    chopped
15ml/1 tbsp finely shredded
    fresh root ginger
30ml/2 tbsp fish sauce
5ml/1 tsp ground star anise
5ml/1 tsp five-spice powder
15ml/1 tbsp oyster sauce
4 spring onions (scallions),
    green parts only, shredded
a small handful of sweet basil
    leaves
a small handful of mint leaves
steamed rice, to serve

Heat a wok over a medium-high heat and add the oil. When hot, add the squash and carrots. Stir-fry for 2–3 minutes, reduce the heat, cover and cook for 5 minutes, until just tender.

Place the beef between 2 sheets of clear film or plastic wrap and beat, with a rolling pin, until thin. Cut into thin strips.

Meanwhile, in a separate wok, add the soy sauce, sugar, chilli, ginger, fish sauce, star anise, five-spice powder and oyster sauce. Cook over a medium heat for 3–4 minutes.

Add the beef strips to the wok and cook over a high heat for 3–4 minutes. Remove from the heat, add the squash, carrots, and spring onion tops and herbs. Serve with steamed rice.

BEEF KEBABS WITH CHESTNUT PURÉE

These spicy Moroccan kebabs are perfect under the grill or on the barbecue. They are complemented by an unusual spicy chestnut purée that makes a good FODMAP-free hummus, which can also be served with crudités.

FODMAP TYPE: Lactose
NUTRITIONAL CONTENT:
Energy 358kcal/1496kJ;
Protein 21g; Carbohydrate 13g, of which sugars 3g; Fat 26g, of which saturates 9g; Cholesterol 61mg; Calcium 115mg; Fibre 2g; Sodium 133mg

Meat

SERVES 6

500g/1¼lb finely minced (ground) beef
10ml/2 tsp ground cumin
10ml/2 tsp ground coriander
10ml/2 tsp paprika
4ml/¾ tsp cayenne pepper
5ml/1 tsp salt
small bunch of flat leaf parsley, finely chopped
small bunch of fresh coriander (cilantro), finely chopped

For the chestnut purée
200g/7oz/1½ cups vacuum-packed shelled chestnuts
50ml/2fl oz/¼ cup olive oil
juice of 1 lemon
5ml/1 tsp cumin seeds
30ml/2 tbsp light tahini
60ml/4 tbsp thick Greek (US strained plain) yogurt
salt and ground black pepper

Mix the beef with all the other ingredients. Knead well, then pulse until smooth in a food processor. Place in a dish, cover and set aside for 1 hour. Preheat the oven to 200°C/400°F/Gas 6.

In a food processor, process the chestnuts with the olive oil, lemon juice, garlic, cumin seeds, tahini and yogurt until smooth. Season, tip into a bowl and set aside.

Divide the meat mixture into six portions and mould each on to a metal skewer.

Heat the grill (broiler) on the hottest setting and cook the kebabs for 4–5 minutes on each side. Serve hot, together with the chestnut purée.

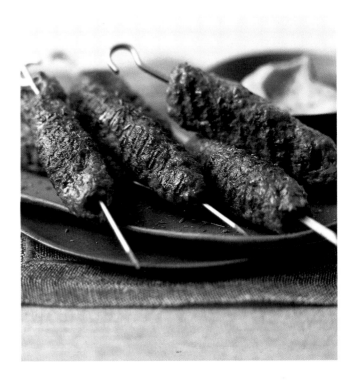

BEEF PIE WITH A POTATO CRUST

This recipe is a variation on traditional cottage pie but incorporates fennel, cheeses and a splash of flavoursome wine. Delicately served in individual ramekins, you can of course bake it in a single ovenproof dish if you prefer.

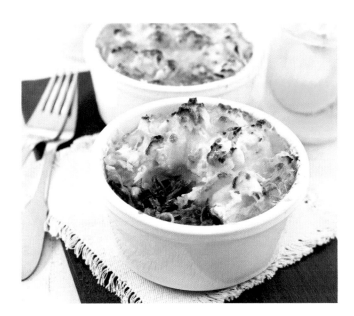

FODMAP TYPE: Lactose
NUTRITIONAL CONTENT:
Energy 859kcal/3591kJ; Protein 29g; Carbohydrate 23g, of which sugars 5g; Fat 70g, of which saturates 38g; Cholesterol 216mg; Calcium 293mg; Fibre 3g; Sodium 685mg

SERVES 4

Meat

500g/1¼lb potatoes, peeled and cooked in salted boiling water until tender
15ml/1 tbsp butter
200ml/7fl oz/scant 1 cup double (heavy) cream
30ml/2 tbsp vegetable oil
115g/4 oz chopped fennel
350g/12oz minced (ground) beef
1 large tomato, peeled, seeded and diced
15g/½oz/¼ cup finely chopped fresh parsley
200ml/7fl oz/scant 1 cup white wine
75g/3oz cream cheese
115g/4oz Cheddar or Gouda cheese, grated
salt and ground black pepper

Drain the cooked potato and mash thoroughly with the butter and cream. Season with salt and pepper to taste.

Heat the oil in a large frying pan, add the fennel and fry for a couple of minutes. Add the beef and fry until completely browned, then add the diced tomato and parsley and cook for another 3–4 minutes.

Add the wine, season, and simmer on a medium heat until the wine has evaporated. Preheat the oven to 190°C/375°F/Gas 5.

To assemble each pie, place a layer of beef in four large ramekins. Cover the meat with a layer of mash, smoothing it to the sides. Top with little lumps of cream cheese, and finally a sprinkling of grated Cheddar or Gouda cheese.

Bake in the oven for 10-15 minutes until the cheese melts and starts to bubble, and serve hot.

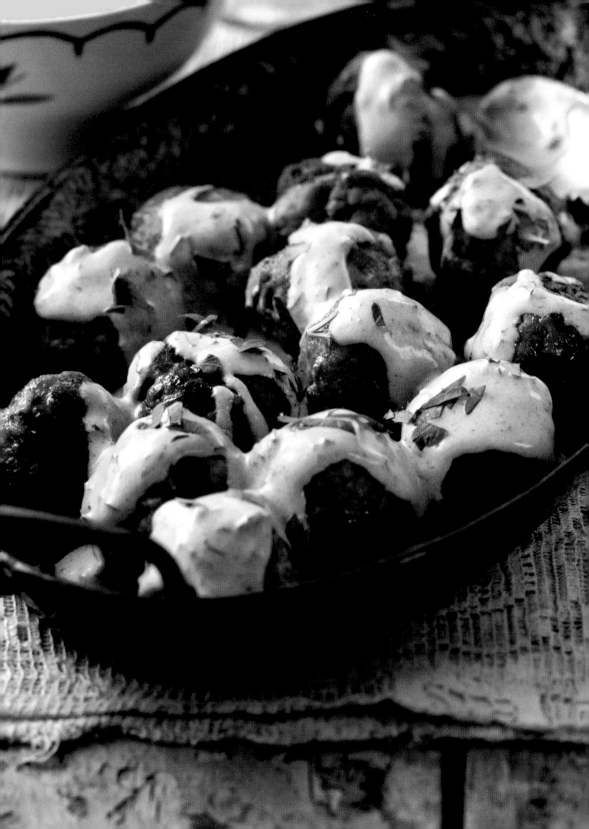

VENISON MEATBALLS

Often thought of as a healthier alternative to beef, venison is a lean but flavoursome meat that is lightened here with the addition of some pork. Serve with mashed potatoes and your favourite low-FODMAP vegetables.

Put the minced venison and minced pork in a bowl and season with salt, pepper and a pinch of asafoetida.

Add the oats, oregano and egg to the bowl, and with your hands, mix them well.

Using your hands again, shape the meat mixture into about 12 meatballs the size of golf balls. If you moisten your hands with a little water first it prevents the mixture from sticking.

When all the balls have been made, roll them in the flour so that they are coated all over.

Add the olive oil to a frying pan, heat the oil and fry the meatballs over a medium heat for 12–15 minutes, turning to cook evenly. Remove from the pan and keep warm.

Add the paprika to the frying pan and stir it into the meat juices, then pour in the chicken stock. Bring to the boil, then simmer until the sauce is reduced by half.

Add the sour cream to the pan and heat until just simmering. Stir in most of the chopped herbs. Pour the sauce over the meatballs, garnish with the remaining herbs and serve.

FODMAP TYPE: Lactose
NUTRITIONAL CONTENT:
Energy 316kcal/1321kJ;
Protein 36g; Carbohydrate 8g,
of which sugars 1g; Fat 16g, of
which saturates 4g; Cholesterol
137mg; Calcium 40mg; Fibre 1g;
Sodium 614mg

Meat

400g/14oz coarsely minced
  (ground) venison
200g/7oz minced (ground) pork
pinch of asafoetida
25g/1oz oats
5–6 oregano sprigs, finely
  chopped
1 egg, beaten
45ml/3 tbsp wheat-free flour,
  for dusting
60ml/4 tbsp olive oil, for frying
5ml/1 tsp sweet paprika
100ml/3½fl oz/scant ½ cup
  onion-free chicken stock
45ml/3 tbsp sour cream
a handful of fresh herbs,
  chopped
salt and ground black pepper

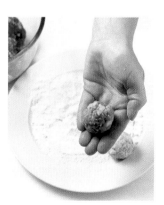
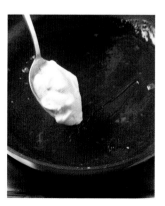

ROASTED LEG OF LAMB WITH RICE

This is a Lebanese-inspired lamb dish served with spicy pinenut and lamb-laced rice. Served with some lightly-sautéed colourful vegetables such as aubergine, courgette and pepper, this would be an impressive centrepiece for a family meal.

FODMAP TYPE: Nil
NUTRITIONAL CONTENT:
Energy 726kcal/3035kJ;
Protein 34g; Carbohydrate 12g,
of which sugars 4g; Fat 61g, of
which saturates 17g; Cholesterol
130mg; Calcium 51mg; Fibre 1g;
Sodium 335mg

Meat

SERVES 6

1kg/2¼lb leg of lamb
2 carrots, peeled and chopped
1 red (bell) pepper, chopped
30–45ml/2–3 tbsp olive oil
a little red wine
sea salt and ground black
    pepper

For the rice
15ml/1 tbsp olive oil plus a
    knob of butter
30ml/2 tbsp pine nuts
10ml/2 tsp ground cinnamon
100g/3¾oz/½ cup lean minced
    (ground) lamb
250g/9oz/1¼ cups long grain
    rice, well rinsed and drained

Preheat the oven to 200°C/400°F/Gas 6. Rub the lamb with salt and pepper and place in a roasting pan with the carrots and red pepper, and drizzle the oil over. Add 300ml/½ pint/1¼ cups water, cover with foil and roast in the oven for 50 minutes.

Meanwhile, prepare the rice. Heat the olive oil with the butter in a heavy pan and add the pine nuts. Cook, stirring, until they begin to colour, then add the cinnamon and minced lamb. Cook for 2–3 minutes, then stir in the rice.

Add 500ml/17fl oz/generous 2 cups water to the pan, season with salt and pepper, and bring to the boil. Reduce the heat and simmer for 15 minutes, until the water has been absorbed. Turn off the heat, cover with a clean dish towel, followed by the lid, and leave for 10–15 minutes.

Take the lamb out of the oven and remove the foil. Baste, then return to the oven, uncovered, for a further 15 minutes. Remove from the oven, and leave to rest.

Strain the juices from the pan and whizz in a blender or food processor with the carrots, red pepper and a dash of wine, to make the gravy. Reheat and transfer to a jug or pitcher.

Spoon some of the rice on to a serving dish to make a bed for the lamb. Place the lamb on top of the rice and spoon the rest of the rice around it. Carve and serve with the gravy.

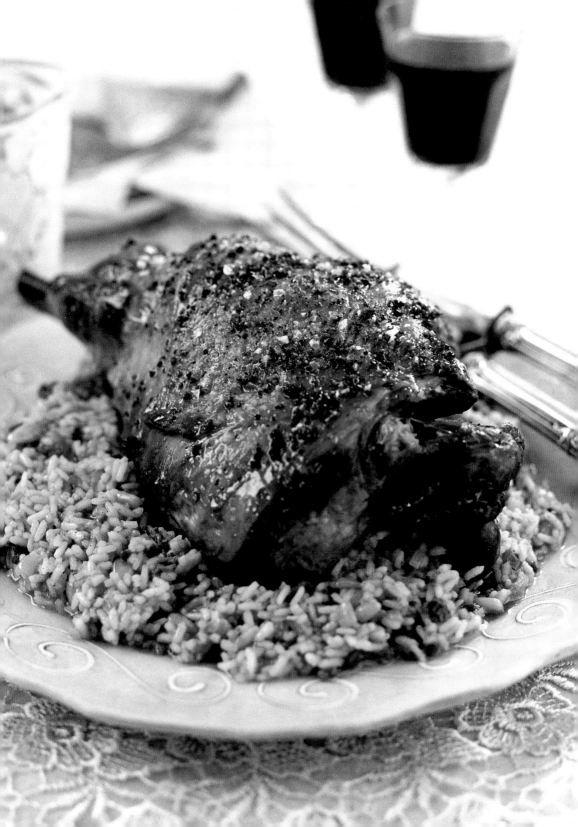

SPICED PORK KEBABS

These FODMAP-free, feisty kebabs can be served as part of a tapas course, or as a main meal with corn tortillas and a fresh, crisp salad. Grinding the seeds releases precious flavours, which are safely captured in lemon juice and oil.

FODMAP TYPE: Nil
NUTRITIONAL CONTENT:
Energy 464kcal/1940kJ;
Protein 55g Carbohydrate 0g,
of which sugars 0g; Fat 28g, of
which saturates 3g; Cholesterol
0mg; Calcium 17mg; Fibre 0g;
Sodium 590mg

SERVES 2

2.5ml/½ tsp cumin seeds
2.5ml/½ tsp coriander seeds
5ml/1 tsp paprika
2.5ml/½ tsp dried oregano
15ml/1 tbsp lemon juice
45ml/3 tbsp olive oil
500g/1¼lb lean pork
salt and ground black pepper

Grind the cumin and coriander seeds in a mortar and add a pinch of salt. Add the paprika and oregano and mix in the lemon juice. Stir in the oil.

Cut the pork into cubes, then push the pieces on to wooden skewers that have been soaked in cold water for 10 minutes. Put the skewers in a shallow dish, pour over the marinade and turn to coat. Leave to marinate in a cool place for 2 hours, turning occasionally.

Preheat the grill (broiler) to high, and line the grill pan with foil. Spread the kebabs out in a row and place under the grill, close to the heat. Cook for about 3 minutes on each side, spooning the juices over when you turn them, until cooked through. Sprinkle with salt and pepper, and serve at once.

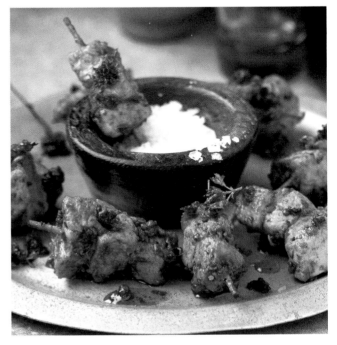

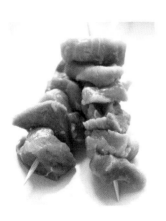

PAPRIKA PORK

This East European-inspired casserole is a handy one to prepare for a slow cooker. It is characteristically sweet and peppery, and is traditionally served with a spoonful of sour cream and boiled rice.

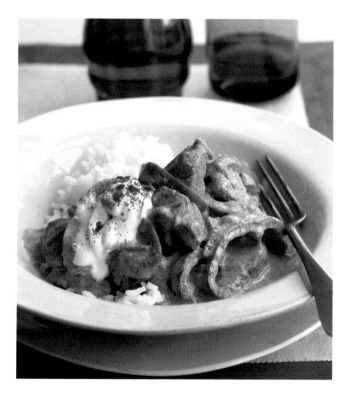

FODMAP TYPE: Lactose
NUTRITIONAL CONTENT:
Energy 436kcal/1119kJ;
Protein 47g; Carbohydrate 6g;
of which sugars 6g; Fat 25g, of
which saturates 7g; Cholesterol
26mg; Calcium 55mg; Fibre 2g;
Sodium 324mg

SERVES 4

Meat

2 pork fillets (tenderloins),
   about 400g/14oz each
45ml/3 tbsp vegetable oil
7.5ml/1½ tsp sweet paprika,
   plus extra to garnish
2 green (bell) peppers, thinly
   sliced into rings
1 tomato, chopped
175ml/6fl oz/¾ cup sour cream,
   plus extra to serve
salt and ground black pepper
boiled rice, to serve

Dice the pork into 3cm/1¼in cubes.

Heat the oil in a flameproof casserole over medium heat and stir in the paprika, then add 100ml/3½fl oz/scant ½ cup water. Return to the heat and simmer for 2–3 minutes.

Add the meat to the casserole and season well. Cover and simmer for 30–40 minutes until the sauce has reduced and the meat is tender. Add the sliced peppers and tomato, and cook for a further 5–6 minutes.

Stir in the sour cream and heat through. Serve with plain boiled rice and a dollop of sour cream sprinkled with paprika.

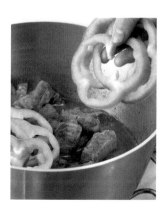

PORK AND CRANBERRY MEATLOAF

This version of the much-loved meatloaf comes from Eastern Europe and is a meal in itself, with sustaining meat, eggs and vegetables served with a herby mayonnaise. Festive cranberries also make it suitable for a Christmas supper.

Meat

FODMAP TYPE: Lactose
NUTRITIONAL CONTENT:
Energy 393kcal/1643kJ;
Protein 43g; Carbohydrate 13g;
of which sugars 8g; Fat 19g, of
which saturates 3g; Cholesterol
172mg; Calcium 39mg; Fibre 1g;
Sodium 111mg

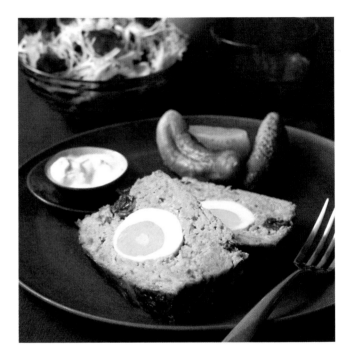

SERVES 6

15ml/1 tbsp vegetable oil, plus
    extra for greasing
green parts of 6 spring onions
    (scallions), finely sliced
1kg/2½lb/5 cups minced
    (ground) pork
2 small eggs, beaten
25g/1oz oats
60ml/4 tbsp frozen or fresh
    cranberries
3 hard-boiled eggs, peeled
salt and ground black pepper
gherkins and green salad,
    to serve

For the sauce
60ml/4 tbsp sour cream
30ml/2 tbsp mayonnaise
5ml/1 tsp finely chopped fresh
    dill
5ml/1 tsp mild mustard
2.5ml/½ tsp sugar

Pour the oil into a pan and add the spring onion tops, fry on a medium heat until soft, then set aside to cool.

Put the pork into a large bowl, with the beaten eggs, oats and cranberries. Add plenty of salt and pepper then combine gently.

Preheat the oven to 180°C/350°F/Gas 4 and lightly oil a 1 litre/1¾ pint/4 cup loaf tin (pan). Spread half the meat mixture in the tin then arrange the hard-boiled eggs on top, in a row down the centre. Cover with the remaining meat mixture. Brush with a little oil and cook in the oven for about 1 hour.

To make the sauce, put all the ingredients in a bowl, season and mix well. Serve the meat loaf warm or cold, accompanied by the dill sauce, gherkins and a green salad.

BRAISED CHINESE-STYLE PORK

This is a classic wok recipe that will bubble away by itself, leaving you with some relaxing time before enjoying with rice and steamed greens. Make sure any stock you use doesn't contain onion or garlic, or replace with water.

Place the pork in a wok or large pan and pour over water to cover. Bring the water to the boil. Cover, reduce the heat and cook gently for 30 minutes. Drain the pork and return to the wok with the stock, and add all the other ingredients.

Add enough water to just cover the pork belly pieces, and cook on a high heat until the mixture comes to a boil.

Cover the wok tightly with a lid, then reduce the heat to low and cook gently for 1½ hours, stirring occasionally to ensure the pork doesn't stick to the base of the wok.

Uncover the wok and simmer for another 30 minutes, until all the liquid has evaporated. Serve with steamed greens and rice.

FODMAP TYPE: Nil
NUTRITIONAL CONTENT:
Energy 540kcal/2257kJ;
Protein 40g; Carbohydrate 6g,
of which sugars 6g; Fat 41g, of
which saturates 15g; Cholesterol
142mg; Calcium 29mg; Fibre 0g;
Sodium 1695mg

SERVES 4

Meat

800g/1¾lb pork belly, trimmed
    and cut into 12 pieces
400ml/14fl oz/1⅔ cups onion-
    free beef stock
75ml/5 tbsp soy sauce
finely grated zest and juice of
    1 large orange
15ml/1 tbsp finely shredded
    fresh root ginger
15ml/1 tbsp hot chilli powder
15ml/1 tbsp muscovado
    (molasses) sugar
3 cinnamon sticks
3 cloves
10 black peppercorns
2–3 star anise
steamed greens and rice,
    to serve

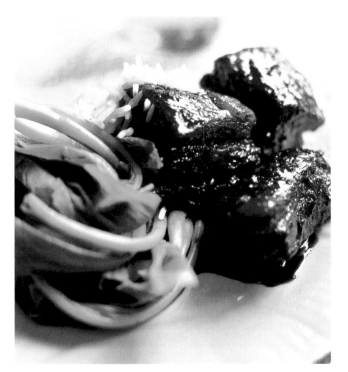

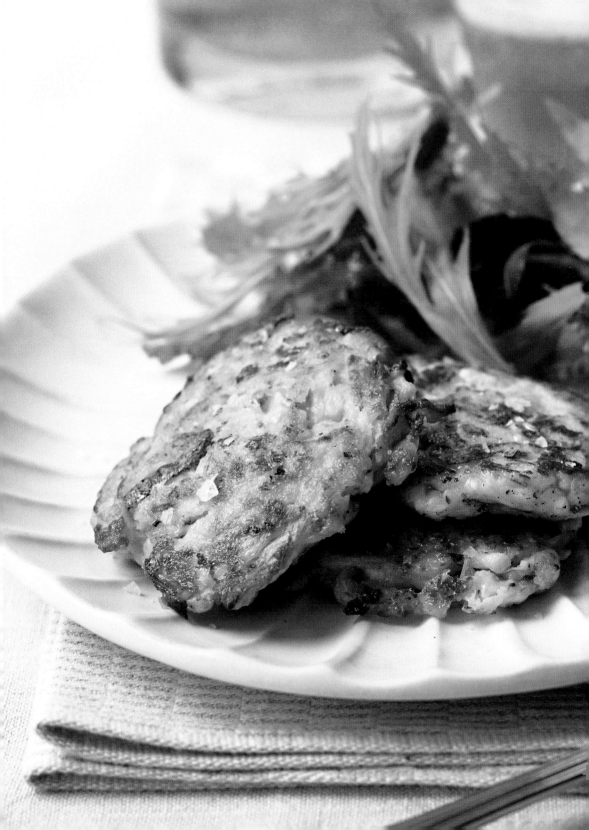

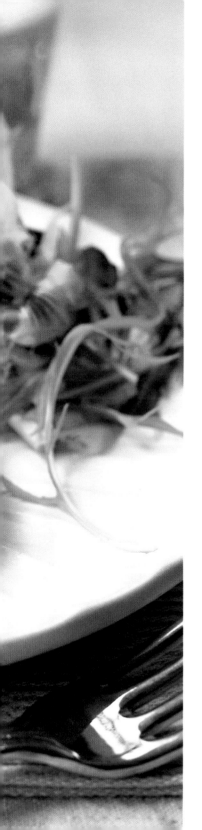

VEGETABLE DISHES

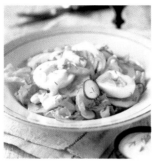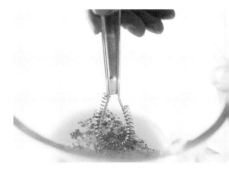

Eating enough fruit and vegetables on a low-FODMAP diet can be tricky, but you'll see from the vibrant recipes in this chapter, for both vegetarian main dishes and accompaniments, that there's still plenty of scope for fresh ideas and variety.

THAI YELLOW VEGETABLE CURRY

Ready-made Thai curry paste contains onion and garlic, but this recipe gives an onion and garlic-free blend of fragrant spices that still creates an authentic curry. Any left-over paste can be stored in the refrigerator.

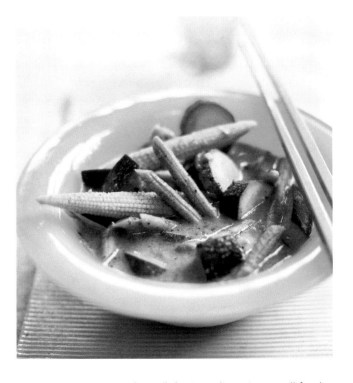

FODMAP TYPE: Polyol (Sorbitol)
NUTRITIONAL CONTENT:
Energy 300kcal/1254kJ;
Protein 6g; Carbohydrate 14g,
of which sugars 13g; Fat 25g, of
which saturates 16g; Cholesterol
0mg; Calcium 72mg; Fibre 4g;
Sodium 783mg

Vegetable Dishes

SERVES 4

30ml/2 tbsp sunflower oil
200ml/7fl oz/scant 1 cup
   coconut cream
300ml/½ pint/1¼ cups coconut
   milk
150ml/¼ pint/⅔ cup onion-free
   vegetable stock (see page 38)
200g/7oz green beans, cut into
   2cm/¾in lengths
200g/7oz baby corn
4 baby courgettes (zucchini),
   sliced
1 small aubergine (eggplant),
   cubed or sliced
10ml/2 tsp palm sugar (jaggery)
salt, to taste

For the yellow curry paste
10ml/2 tsp hot chilli powder
10ml/2 tsp ground coriander
10ml/2 tsp ground cumin
5ml/1 tsp turmeric
30ml/2 tbsp finely chopped
   lemon grass
5ml/1 tsp grated lime zest

Make the curry paste. Place all the ingredients in a small food processor and blend with 30–45ml/2–3 tbsp of cold water to make a smooth paste. Add a little more water if the paste seems too dry.

Heat a large wok over a medium heat and add the sunflower oil. When hot add 30–45ml/2–3 tbsp of the curry paste and stir-fry for 1–2 minutes. Add the coconut cream and cook gently for 8–10 minutes, or until the mixture starts to separate.

Add the coconut milk, stock and vegetables and cook gently for 8–10 minutes, until the vegetables are just tender. Stir in the palm sugar, add salt to taste, and serve in bowls.

EGG, POTATO AND GREEN PEA CURRY

This vegetarian main dish includes hard-boiled eggs that are coated in turmeric and chilli, forming a fragrant, coloured crust. Cooked with sustaining potatoes and peas, it culminates in a nutritious one-pot supper.

Make four small slits in each egg. Heat the oil over a low heat and add 1.5ml/¼ tsp each of the turmeric and chilli powder, followed by the whole eggs. Stir-fry the eggs until they develop a light golden crust all over. Remove and set aside.

Add the potatoes to the same oil and increase the heat to medium. Stir-fry until they also develop a light golden crust. Remove and drain on kitchen paper. Reduce the heat to low and add the cinnamon, cardamom, cloves and bay leaves and fry for a few seconds. Add the ground coriander and cumin and remaining turmeric and chilli powder. Stir-fry for 1 minute, then add the tomato and continue to cook for 1–2 minutes.

Add the potatoes, salt and sugar, and 250ml/8fl oz/1 cup water. Bring to the boil, cover, and reduce the heat to low. Cook until the potatoes are tender. Add the peas and cook for 5–6 minutes longer. Add the eggs, stir in the garam masala and serve.

FODMAP TYPE: GOS
NUTRITIONAL CONTENT:
Energy 161kcal/673kJ;
Protein 9g; Carbohydrate 17g,
of which sugars 2g; Fat 7g, of
which saturates 2g; Cholesterol
223mg; Calcium 57mg; Fibre 2g;
Sodium 377mg

SERVES 4　　127

4 hard-boiled eggs, shelled
60ml/4 tbsp sunflower oil
2.5ml/½ tsp ground turmeric
2.5ml/½ tsp chilli powder
350g/12oz potatoes, peeled,
　　quartered, washed and dried
2.5cm/1in cinnamon stick
4 green cardamom pods,
　　bruised
4 cloves
2 bay leaves
5ml/1 tsp ground coriander
2.5ml/½ tsp ground cumin
1 fresh tomato, skinned and
　　chopped
5ml/1 tsp salt or to taste
2.5ml/½ tsp sugar
50g/2oz/½ cup frozen peas
2.5ml/½ tsp garam masala

Vegetable Dishes

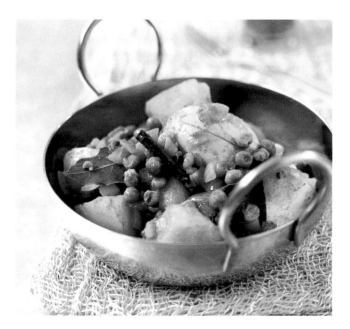

AUBERGINE PILAFF WITH CINNAMON AND MINT

This Middle-Eastern inspired recipe includes a wonderfully rustic blend of dried fruit, seeds and brightly coloured vegetables. It is eye-catching either served as a side dish, or topped with freshly fried halloumi, meat or fish.

Vegetable Dishes

FODMAP TYPE: Fructans
NUTRITIONAL CONTENT:
Energy 317kcal/1325kJ;
Protein 5g; Carbohydrate 26g,
of which sugars 12g; Fat 22g, of
which saturates 2g; Cholesterol
0mg; Calcium 173mg; Fibre 3g;
Sodium 274mg

SERVES 6

2 large aubergines (eggplants)
30–45ml/2–3 tbsp olive oil
30–45ml/2–3 tbsp pine nuts
5ml/1 tsp coriander seeds
30ml/2 tbsp currants, soaked in
    warm water for 5–10
    minutes and drained
10–15ml/2–3 tsp sugar
15–30ml/1–2 tbsp cinnamon
15–30ml/1–2 tbsp dried mint
1 small bunch of fresh dill,
    finely chopped
3 tomatoes, skinned, seeded
    and finely chopped
350g/12oz/generous 1¾ cups
    long or short grain rice, well
    rinsed and drained
sunflower oil, for frying
juice of ½ lemon
salt and ground black pepper
fresh mint sprigs and lemon
    wedges, to serve

Peel the aubergines lengthways in stripes. Quarter them lengthways, then slice each quarter into bitesize chunks and place in a bowl of salted water. Cover with a plate to keep them submerged, and leave to soak for at least 30 minutes.

Meanwhile, heat the oil in a heavy pan, stir in the pine nuts and cook until golden. Stir in the coriander seeds, currants, sugar, cinnamon, mint and dill, then stir in the tomatoes.

Stir in the rice, then pour in 900ml/1½ pints/3¾ cups water, season with salt and pepper and bring to the boil. Lower the heat and partially cover the pan, then simmer for 10–12 minutes, until almost all of the water has been absorbed. Turn off the heat, cover the pan with a dish towel and press the lid tightly on top. Leave the rice to steam for about 15 minutes.

Heat a good glug of sunflower oil in a wok or frying pan. Drain the aubergines and squeeze them dry, then toss them in batches in the oil, for a few minutes at a time. When they are golden brown, lift out and drain on kitchen paper.

Transfer the rice to a serving bowl and toss the aubergine chunks through it with the lemon juice. Garnish with mint sprigs and serve with lemon wedges for squeezing.

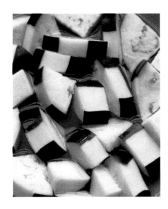
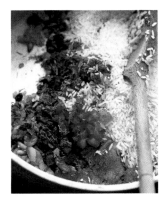

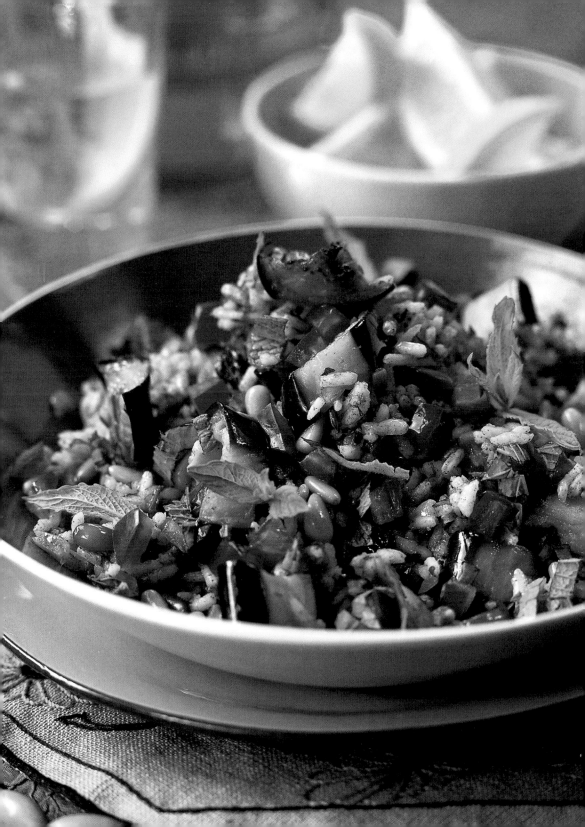

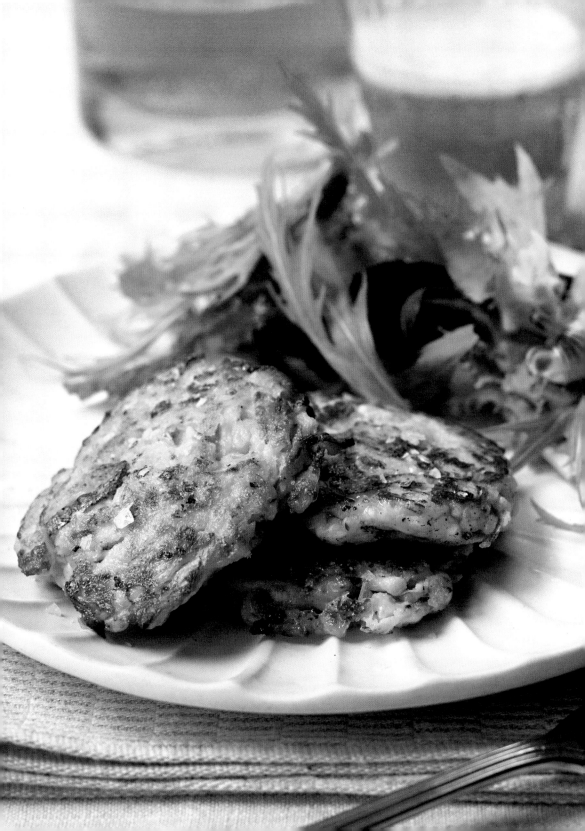

COURGETTE AND FETA FRITTERS

These delicious, moist morsels of FODMAP-friendly courgette and feta can be savoured as a light lunch or a vegetable accompaniment. Prepare these in advance if easier, they will crisp up again nicely in a warm oven.

Lay a clean dish towel on the work surface and grate the courgettes on to it. Gather up the corners of the towel so that the grated courgettes are pushed into a ball inside the towel, then use your hands to squeeze the excess liquid out.

Heat the oil in a frying pan, and gently fry the sliced spring onion tops until soft. Transfer to a large bowl.

In a separate bowl, beat the egg with the cornflour until well blended. Season with pepper and add to the spring onion tops with the grated courgettes and mint. Fold the crumbled feta cheese into the mixture and add a little salt if needed.

Add a little olive oil to a heavy, non-stick frying pan and spoon in three or four tablespoons of the courgette mixture, to make a few fritters at a time.

Cook the fritters on one side for 3–4 minutes, or until set and lightly browned, then turn over and cook the other side for 3–4 minutes, or until browned.

Drain the fritters on kitchen paper and keep them warm while you cook the remaining mixture. Serve warm, with a fresh green salad if you wish.

FODMAP TYPE: Nil
NUTRITIONAL CONTENT:
Energy 291kcal/1216kJ;
Protein 10g; Carbohydrate 13g,
of which sugars 3g; Fat 22g, of
which saturates 8g; Cholesterol
85mg; Calcium 183mg; Fibre 1g;
Sodium 567mg

SERVES 4

131

Vegetable Dishes

450g/1lb courgettes (zucchini),
30ml/2 tbsp olive oil
6 spring onion (scallions) green
   tops only, thinly sliced
1 large (US extra large) egg
45ml/3 tbsp cornflour
   (cornstarch)
1 small bunch mint, leaves
   finely chopped
150g/5oz feta cheese, crumbled
olive oil, for shallow-frying
salt and ground black pepper
green salad, to serve

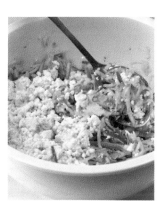

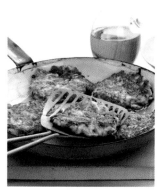

ROASTED PEPPERS WITH HALLOUMI AND PINE NUTS

Halloumi cheese is a great cheese to cook, as its distinct saltiness adds flavour and its firmness withstands high temperatures. It is perfect roasted as in this classic recipe. Serves two with a green salad for a light lunch, or four as an appetizer.

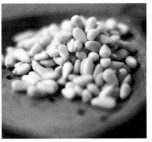

SERVES 2

4 red and 2 orange or yellow
   (bell) peppers
60ml/4 tbsp garlic-infused or
   herb olive oil
250g/9oz halloumi cheese
50g/2oz/½ cup pine nuts

VARIATION You could replace the halloumi cheese with 115g/4oz of feta cheese, if you prefer.

Preheat the oven to 220°C/425°F/Gas 7. Halve the red peppers, leaving the stalks intact, and discard the seeds. Seed and coarsely chop the orange or yellow peppers.

Place the red pepper halves on a baking sheet and fill with the chopped peppers. Drizzle with half the garlic or herb olive oil and bake for 25 minutes, until the edges of the peppers are beginning to char.

Dice the cheese and tuck in among the chopped peppers. Sprinkle with the pine nuts and drizzle with the remaining oil. Bake for a further 15 minutes, until well browned. Serve warm.

FODMAP TYPE: Lactose
NUTRITIONAL CONTENT:
Energy 443kcal/1852kJ;
Protein 17g; Carbohydrate 8g,
of which sugars 7g; Fat 38g, of
which saturates 13g; Cholesterol
0mg; Calcium 21mg; Fibre 5g;
Sodium 642mg

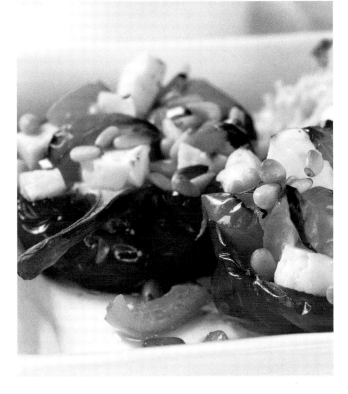

RADICCHIO FRITTATA

The distinctive red and white leaves of radicchio lettuce, an Italian relative of chicory, is often used in salads to provide a distinct bitterness. In this light cream-laced frittata, it retains some crunchy bite.

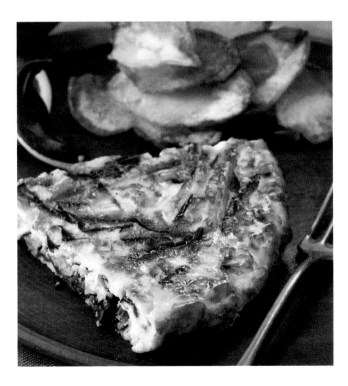

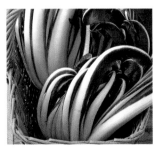

Vegetable Dishes

SERVES 4

90ml/6 tbsp single (light) cream
250g/9oz/3 cups freshly grated
  Parmesan cheese
5 eggs, beaten
45ml/3 tbsp olive oil
25g/1oz/2 tbsp unsalted butter
5 heads of radicchio, or red
  endive, sliced into strips
sea salt and ground black
  pepper
fried potatoes, to serve

VARIATION Replace the radicchio with 4 handfuls of sliced Swiss chard.

FODMAP TYPE: Lactose
NUTRITIONAL CONTENT:
Energy 555kcal/2320kJ;
Protein 34g; Carbohydrate 1g,
of which sugars 1g; Fat 46g, of
which saturates 22g; Cholesterol
332mg; Calcium 833mg; Fibre
1g; Sodium 518mg

Whisk the cream with the Parmesan cheese and eggs, then season with salt. Heat the oil and butter in a large frying pan.

Mix the radicchio or red endive into the egg mixture, then pour it into the hot pan. Shake the pan to flatten and even out the mixture, then cook until the underside is browned and firm.

Turn over the frittata by covering the pan with a large plate and then overturning the pan, then slide the frittata (uncooked side down) back into the hot pan.

Continue to cook the frittata until golden brown and firm on the underside. Slide out on to a clean platter and serve warm, with some fried potatoes and extra radicchio, if you like.

STUFFED COURGETTES

Pomegranate seeds have been used medicinally for thousands of years; they are also high in fibre and vitamins A, C and E, add a beautiful decorative red to the dish, and most important of all, have an acceptable FODMAP content.

FODMAP TYPE: Fructans
NUTRITIONAL CONTENT:
Energy 464kcal/1940kJ;
Protein 13g Carbohydrate 19g,
of which sugars 9g; Fat 38g, of
which saturates 6g; Cholesterol
20mg; Calcium 180mg; Fibre 4g;
Sodium 471mg

SERVES 4

115g/4oz/1 cup pine nuts
8 pale-green courgettes
  (zucchini)
30ml/2 tbsp olive oil, plus extra
  for drizzling
2.5ml/½ tsp ground allspice
2.5ml/½ tsp ground cinnamon
185g/6½oz/scant 1 cup long
  grain rice
seeds of 1 pomegranate
60ml/4 tbsp chopped fresh
  parsley
salt and ground black pepper
115g/4oz feta cheese, to serve

VARIATION This filling is also delicious used as a stuffing for green (bell) peppers, topped with Parmesan rather than feta.

Put the pine nuts in a dry pan and toast over medium-high heat, tossing regularly, for 1–2 minutes, or until golden brown. Set aside. Halve the courgettes lengthways. Using a small sharp knife, carefully hollow them out, removing all the seed pulp from the centre.

To make the stuffing, heat the olive oil in a large sauté pan and add the allspice and cinnamon. Sauté for a few seconds, then add the rice and cook for a further 2 minutes, making sure that the rice grains are well coated with the spice mixture.

Add 150ml/¼ pint/⅔ cup water and season with salt and pepper, then cook until the rice is al dente: tender with a bite in the centre. Remove from the heat, add the pine nuts, pomegranate seeds and parsley, then leave to cool. Preheat the oven to 180°C/350°F/Gas 4.

Fill the courgette halves with the stuffing and put into an ovenproof dish. Drizzle with a little olive oil and add about 100ml/3½fl oz/scant ½ cup water to the dish.

Bake uncovered for about 30 minutes, or until tender, basting occasionally with the pan juices. Serve warm with feta cheese crumbled over the top.

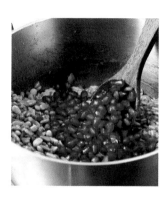

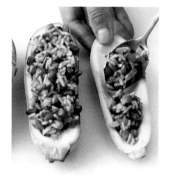

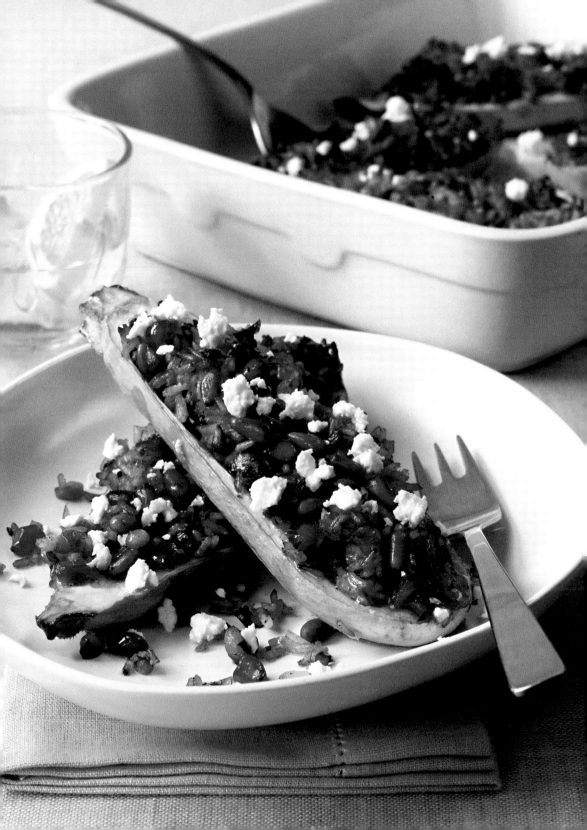

POTATO AND PARSNIP GRATIN

This variation on the classic potato dish uses a mixture of parsnip and potato for a lighter result. Easy to prepare in advance, it can be eaten as a main meal with a selection of salads, or as an accompaniment to roast meat.

FODMAP TYPE: Lactose
NUTRITIONAL CONTENT:
Energy 364kcal/1522kJ;
Protein 12g; Carbohydrate 41g;
of which sugars 11g; Fat 18g, of
which saturates 11g; Cholesterol
46mg; Calcium 231mg; Fibre 6g;
Sodium 178mg

SERVES 4

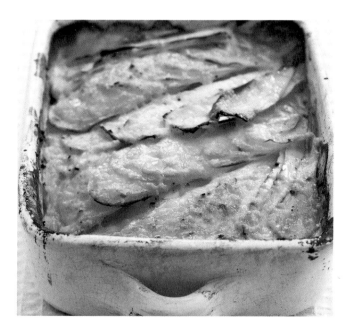

3 large potatoes, total weight about 675g/1½lb, peeled and cut into very thin slices
350g/12oz small- to medium-sized parsnips, peeled and cut into very thin slices
200ml/7fl oz/scant 1 cup single (light) cream
100ml/3½fl oz/scant ½ cup lactose-free milk, eg rice or soya
butter, for greasing
about 5ml/1 tsp freshly grated nutmeg
75g/3oz/¾ cup coarsely grated mature (sharp) Cheddar or Red Leicester cheese
salt and ground black pepper

Cook the sliced potatoes and parsnips in a large pan of salted boiling water for 5 minutes. Drain and cool slightly.

Meanwhile, pour the cream and milk into a heavy pan and bring to the boil over a medium heat. Remove from the heat and leave to stand for about 10 minutes.

Preheat the oven to 180°C/350°F/Gas 4 and lightly butter the bottom and sides of a shallow ovenproof dish. Arrange the potatoes and parsnips in the dish, sprinkling each layer with a little freshly grated nutmeg, salt and ground black pepper.

Pour the liquid into the dish and cover with lightly buttered foil. Cook in the hot oven for 45 minutes. Remove the foil and sprinkle the grated cheese on top. Return to the oven and cook, uncovered, for a further 20–30 minutes, or until the potatoes and parsnips are tender and the top is golden brown.

MINI BAKED POTATOES WITH BLUE CHEESE

These soft little potatoes, laced with sour cream, cheese and chives, make an eye-catching accompaniment to most main dishes. For an impressive appetizer, add a slither of smoked salmon or prosciutto.

Preheat the oven to 180°C/350°F/Gas 4. Wash and dry the potatoes. Pour the oil into a bowl. Add the potatoes and toss to coat well with oil.

Dip the potatoes in the coarse salt to coat lightly. Spread out the potatoes on a baking sheet. Bake for 45–50 minutes until tender. In a bowl, use a fork to mash the blue cheese with the sour cream.

Cut a cross in the top of each cooked potato. Press gently with your fingers to open the potatoes. Top each potato with a dollop of the cheese mixture. It will melt down into the potato nicely. Sprinkle with chives, place on a serving dish and serve hot or at room temperature.

FODMAP TYPE: Lactose
NUTRITIONAL CONTENT:
Energy 300kcal/1254kJ;
Protein 5g; Carbohydrate 25g;
of which sugars 3g; Fat 21g, of
which saturates 7g; Cholesterol
74mg; Calcium 63mg; Fibre 3g;
Sodium 381mg

SERVES 4

20 small new or salad potatoes
60ml/4 tbsp vegetable oil
coarse salt
25g/1oz blue cheese, crumbled
120ml/4fl oz/½ cup sour cream
30ml/2 tbsp chopped fresh
  chives, for sprinkling

Vegetable Dishes

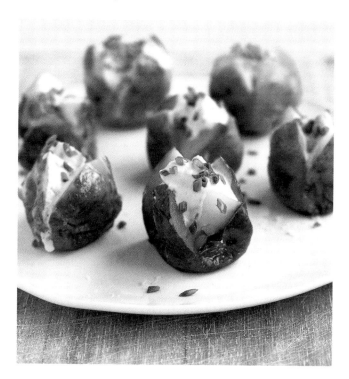

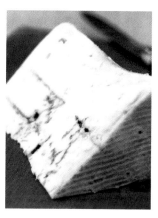

ENDIVE MASH

The slightly bitter leaves of endive, often used in salads, are also delicious cooked with mashed potato. A little milk, as used here, should be acceptable even for those intolerant of lactose, but can easily be substituted if preferred.

FODMAP TYPE: Lactose
NUTRITIONAL CONTENT:
Energy 467kcal/1952kJ;
Protein 23g; Carbohydrate 47g,
of which sugars 5g; Fat 22g, of
which saturates 14g; Cholesterol
57mg; Calcium 540mg; Fibre 9g;
Sodium 848mg

SERVES 4

1kg/2¼lb potatoes, peeled
200g/7oz/1¾ cups mild Gouda
  cheese
25g/1oz/2 tbsp butter
100ml/3½fl oz/scant ½ cup hot
  milk
1kg/2¼lb endive or frisée
  lettuce, cut into thin strips
salt
butter and ground black
  pepper, to serve

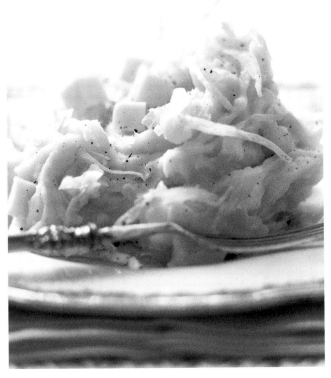

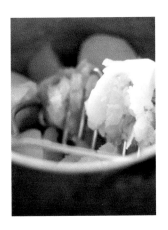

Cook the potatoes in lightly salted boiling water for about 20 minutes, until tender.

Cut the cheese into small dice.

Drain the potatoes, return to the pan and mash with the butter and enough of the hot milk to make a smooth but not thin purée. Add salt to taste.

Stir in the endive or frisée lettuce and then fold in most of the cheese. Serve piping hot in a mound topped with a generous knob (pat) of butter, black pepper and the rest of the cheese.

SPICED POTATO CAKES

French fries or regular potato croquettes will seem very dull after eating these spiced, herby morsels of creamy, mashed potato. Leave the chilli out if you know your constitution is more sensitive to spices.

In a small pan, heat the oil over a medium heat and add the fennel seeds. Allow them to sizzle for a few seconds, then add the chillies and ginger. Stir in the turmeric, coriander leaves and salt, and remove from the heat.

Put the mashed potato in a mixing bowl and add the spice mixture, mix well and add the cornflour and egg. Stir until all the ingredients are well blended.

Heat the oil for deep-frying in a wok or other suitable pan over a medium/high heat. Drop a tiny amount of the potato mixture into the oil to test the temperature, if it sizzles and floats to the top immediately, the oil is the right temperature.

With two spoons, make rough croquette shapes out of the mixture, lowering each one into the hot oil. Fry in batches until browned and drain on kitchen paper.

FODMAP TYPE: Nil
NUTRITIONAL CONTENT:
Energy 235kcal/982kJ;
Protein 4g; Carbohydrate 24g,
of which sugars 1g; Fat 15g, of
which saturates 2g; Cholesterol
59mg; Calcium 23mg; Fibre 2g;
Sodium 527mg

SERVES 4

30ml/2 tbsp vegetable oil
2.5ml/½ tsp fennel seeds
1–2 green chillies, deseeded
   and chopped
10ml/2 tsp ginger purée
2.5ml/½ tsp ground turmeric
30ml/2 tbsp coriander (cilantro)
   leaves, chopped
5ml/1 tsp salt or to taste
450g/1lb potatoes, boiled and
   lightly mashed
15ml/1 tbsp cornflour
   (cornstarch)
1 large egg, beaten
oil for deep frying

Vegetable Dishes

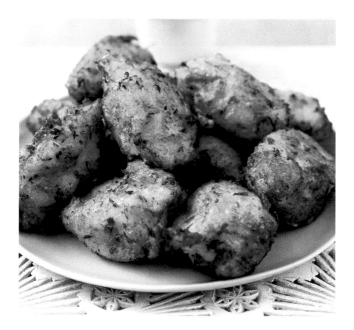

FENNEL WITH PARMESAN

A highly versatile and low-FODMAP vegetable, fennel adds a mild aniseed flavour eaten either cooked or raw. It is matched here with Parmesan to create a side dish that would be perfect served with fish.

FODMAP TYPE: Lactose
NUTRITIONAL CONTENT:
Energy 580kcal/2424kJ; Protein 21g; Carbohydrate 4g, of which sugars 4g; Fat 54g, of which saturates 34g; Cholesterol 145mg; Calcium 617mg; Fibre 5g; Sodium 603mg

Vegetable Dishes

SERVES 4

6 large fennel bulbs (or 8 small ones), trimmed
185g/6½oz/generous ¾ cup unsalted butter, melted
185g/6½oz/generous 2 cups freshly grated Parmesan cheese, plus extra to serve
sea salt and ground black pepper

Boil the whole fennel bulbs in salted water for 30 minutes, or until soft and tender. Drain and cut them lengthways into finger-thick slices.

Preheat the oven to 180°C/350°F/Gas 4. Brush some of the melted butter over the base of an ovenproof dish.

Arrange half the fennel in a layer in the dish and cover with half the melted butter and Parmesan, then a sprinkling of salt and pepper. Repeat with the rest of the ingredients.

Bake for 20 minutes, or until golden, and serve, sprinkled with extra Parmesan.

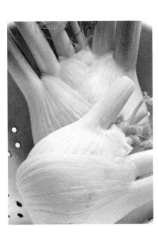

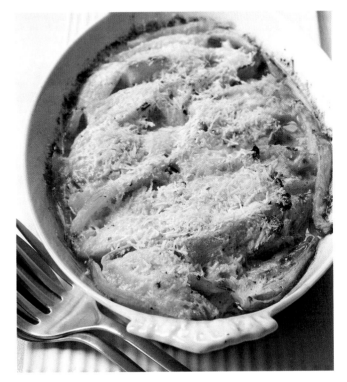

BAKED AUBERGINES WITH MOZZARELLA

Baked mozzarella, encased by delicate, egg-fried aubergine, make up these memorable morsels. Italian inspired, serve them as an appetizer, or light lunch accompanied by polenta or a red pepper salad.

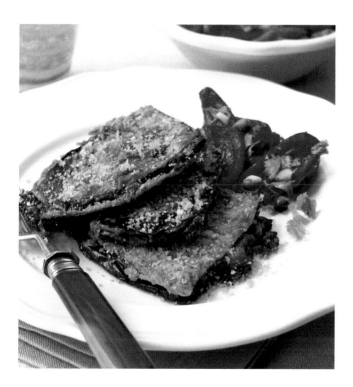

FODMAP TYPE: Lactose
NUTRITIONAL CONTENT:
Energy 238kcal/995kJ;
Protein 11g; Carbohydrate 6g,
of which sugars 2g; Fat 19g, of
which saturates 7g; Cholesterol
89mg; Calcium 228mg; Fibre 2g;
Sodium 430mg

SERVES 6

2 eggs
500g/1¼lb aubergines
  (eggplants)
cornflour (cornstarch),
  for dusting
350ml/12fl oz/1½ cups olive oil
150g/5oz mozzarella cheese,
  thinly sliced
60ml/4 tbsp grated Parmesan
salt and ground black pepper
red (bell) pepper salad, to serve

Vegetable Dishes

Put the eggs in a bowl. Season with salt and pepper and beat them lightly. Coat the aubergine slices lightly in cornflour, then dip each slice into the egg. Heat the oil in a large frying pan.

Fry the floured aubergine slices, in batches if necessary, for 3 minutes on each side, until crisp and golden, then drain on kitchen paper. Preheat the oven to 200°C/400°F/Gas 6.

Arrange half the aubergine slices in a roasting pan. Top each one with a slice of mozzarella. Cover with the remaining fried aubergine slices, pressing together to form sandwiches.

Season with a little salt, sprinkle evenly with the Parmesan and bake for 10 minutes. Serve immediately.

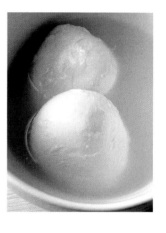

KALE WITH MUSTARD DRESSING

Due to its very high beta-carotene content, together with good iron and antioxidant lutein levels, kale is sometimes deemed a 'superfood'. In this recipe, vinegar and oil form a thick and delicious emulsion with the help of mustard.

FODMAP TYPE: Nil
NUTRITIONAL CONTENT:
Energy 104kcal/435kJ;
Protein 2g; Carbohydrate 1g,
of which sugars 1g; Fat 10g, of
which saturates 1g; Cholesterol
0mg; Calcium 83mg; Fibre 2g;
Sodium 341mg

Wash the kale, drain thoroughly, then trim off the thickest stalks and cut the leaves in two. Steam in a large pan with a sprinkling of water, covered, for 4–5 minutes until wilted.

Whisk the oil into the mustard in a bowl. When it is blended completely, whisk in the white wine vinegar. It should begin to thicken. Season the mustard dressing to taste with sugar, salt and ground black pepper. Toss the kale in the dressing and serve immediately.

SERVES 4

250g/9oz curly kale
45ml/3 tbsp light olive oil
5ml/1 tsp wholegrain mustard
15ml/1 tbsp white wine vinegar
pinch of caster (superfine)
    sugar
salt and ground black pepper

VARIATION Cook Swiss Chard in the same way, and replace the wholegrain mustard with Dijon, if you wish.

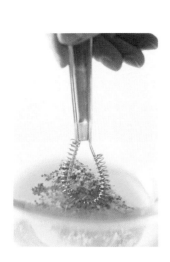

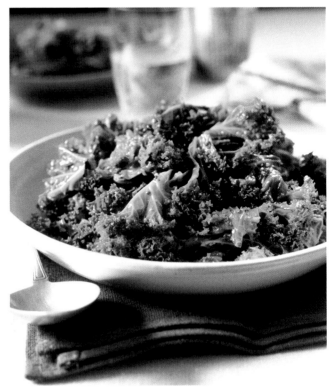

COLESLAW AND BLUE CHEESE

This is a decadent twist on regular coleslaw with a creamy blue cheese and sharp, yogurty dressing. The cabbage type is important as green Savoy cabbage is much higher in FODMAPs than white, so don't be tempted to substitute.

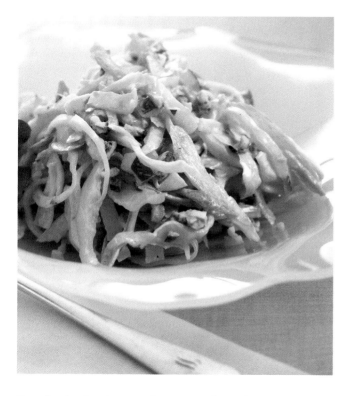

FODMAP TYPE: Polyol (Mannitol)
NUTRITIONAL CONTENT:
Energy 118kcal/493kJ;
Protein 4g; Carbohydrate 6g,
of which sugars 6g; Fat 9g, of
which saturates 3g; Cholesterol
14mg; Calcium 87mg; Fibre 2g;
Sodium 261mg

SERVES 6–8

143

Vegetable Dishes

45ml/3 tbsp mayonnaise
45ml/3 tbsp thick natural
   (plain) yogurt
50g/2oz blue cheese, such as
   Stilton
15ml/1 tbsp lemon juice
500g/1¼lb white cabbage
1 medium carrot
2 small celery sticks
a few radishes
salt and ground black pepper

To make the dressing, put the mayonnaise and yogurt into a large bowl and crumble in the cheese. Stir well, adding a squeeze of lemon juice and seasoning to taste.

Trim and shred the cabbage finely, grate the carrot, cut the celery into very thin slices and chop the radishes.

Add the cabbage, carrot, celery and radishes to the bowl and toss until all the ingredients are well mixed and coated with the dressing.

Cover the bowl and chill in the refrigerator for 2–3 hours or until ready to serve. Stir before serving.

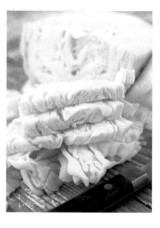

WARM SPRING CABBAGE SALAD

Fresh, spring vegetables are packed full of crispness and flavour, and, due its to sulphur-containing compounds, cabbage also has health benefits. Home-prepared garlic-infused oil is fine, so long as no garlic pieces remain.

FODMAP TYPE: Nil
NUTRITIONAL CONTENT:
Energy 390kcal/1630kJ;
Protein 2g; Carbohydrate 5g,
of which sugars 5g; Fat 40g, of
which saturates 6g; Cholesterol
0mg; Calcium 49mg; Fibre 2g;
Sodium 204mg

Vegetable Dishes

SERVES 6

1 large white or spring cabbage
300ml/½ pint/1¼ cups extra
   virgin olive oil
100ml/3½fl oz/scant ½ cup red
   wine vinegar
3 garlic cloves, slightly crushed
sea salt and ground black
   pepper

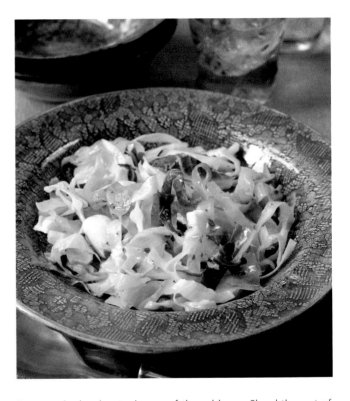

Remove the hard outer leaves of the cabbage. Shred the rest of the cabbage finely and put it into a colander. Rinse it well several times, then drain thoroughly.

Pour the oil and vinegar into a pan over a medium heat. Add the garlic. Heat until sizzling.

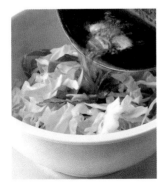

Transfer the shredded cabbage to a salad bowl, then pour over the hot garlic oil. Discard the garlic cloves.

Toss the mixture together. Season with salt and pepper, toss again and cover with a plate to allow it to steam for about 2–3 minutes. Serve while still warm.

LETTUCE AND EGG SALAD

A sweet and sharp dressing offsets the heat of radishes that interestingly are FODMAP-friendly, despite sharing familial roots with broccoli and cauliflower, which are not. This salad is best served crisp and fresh.

First make the dressing so it has time for the flavours to develop. Put the crème fraîche and lemon juice in a small bowl and whisk together. Add the sugar and salt and stir until the sugar is completely dissolved. Set aside.

Remove the shells from the eggs, and cut in half. Cut the lettuce into pieces and put in a serving dish. Peel and finely slice the cucumber, and radishes. Layer the salad by placing the cucumber on top of the shredded lettuce, then the radishes, then the egg halves.

Spoon the dressing over the salad and garnish with chopped fresh dill and sliced spring onion. Serve immediately.

FODMAP TYPE: Lactose
NUTRITIONAL CONTENT:
Energy 260kcal/1087kJ;
Protein 6g; Carbohydrate 8g,
of which sugars 7g; Fat 23g, of
which saturates 14g; Cholesterol
154mg; Calcium 74mg; Fibre 2g;
Sodium 248mg

SERVES 4

Vegetable Dishes

2 eggs, hard-boiled
1 large cos or romaine lettuce, washed and drained
1 cucumber
10 radishes
fresh dill and sliced spring onion (scallion), green tops only, to garnish

For the dressing
200ml/7fl oz/scant 1 cup crème fraîche
juice of 1 lemon
15ml/1 tbsp sugar
pinch of salt

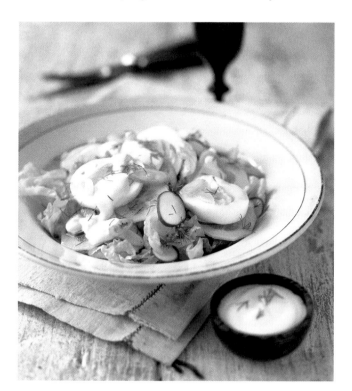

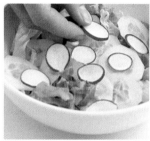

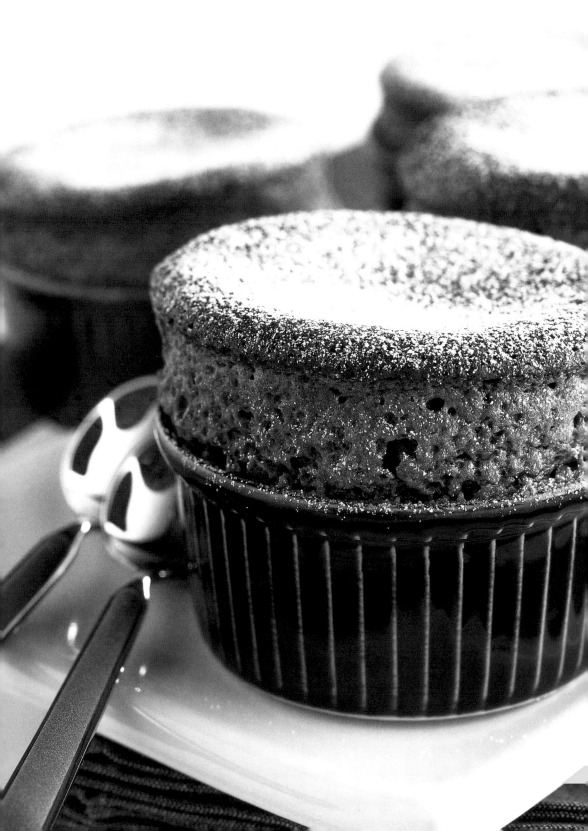

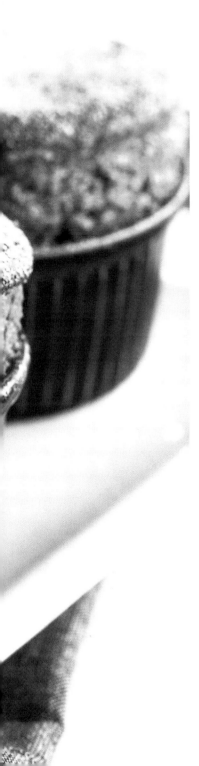

DESSERTS & BAKING

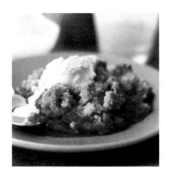 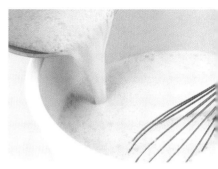

Don't compromise on enjoying sweet treats when on a low-FODMAP diet, but instead make use of wheat-free baking alternatives including ground nuts, oats and polenta. Cream and yogurt also feature, which are fine in the quantities suggested here, and help boost calcium intake. They are complemented with suitable fruits.

LEMON MERINGUE PIE

With a thin pastry crust and a filling thickened with cornflour, this classic English dessert can easily be adapted to a low-FODMAP dish by using wheat-free flour. Best served warm it can also be chilled, although the meringue may soften.

FODMAP TYPE: Nil
NUTRITIONAL CONTENT:
Energy 357kcal/1492kJ;
Protein 3.4g; Carbohydrate 66g,
of which sugars 42g; Fat 12g of
which saturates 6g; Cholesterol
87mg; Calcium 36mg; Fibre 1g;
Sodium 311mg

Desserts & Baking

SERVES 6

For the pastry
115g/4oz/1 cup wheat-free
 plain (all-purpose) flour
pinch of salt
50g/2oz butter, diced

For the filling
50g/2oz/¼ cup cornflour
 (cornstarch)
175g/6oz/¾ cup caster
 (superfine) sugar
finely grated rind and juice of
 2 lemons
2 egg yolks
15g/½oz/1 tbsp butter, diced

For the meringue topping
2 egg whites
75g/3oz/½ cup caster
 (superfine) sugar

To make the pastry, sift the flour and salt into a bowl and add the butter. With the fingertips, lightly rub the butter into the flour until the mixture resembles fine crumbs.

Stir in about 20ml/2 tbsp cold water until the mixture can be gathered together into a smooth ball of dough. (Alternatively make the pastry using a food processor.) Wrap the pastry and chill in the refrigerator for at least 30 minutes. Meanwhile, preheat the oven to 200°C/400°F/Gas 6.

Roll out the pastry on a lightly floured surface and use to line a 20cm/8in flan tin (pie pan). Prick the base with a fork, line with baking parchment or foil and add a layer of baking beans to prevent the pastry rising.

Put the pastry case (pie shell) into the hot oven and cook for 15 minutes. Remove the beans and parchment or foil, return the pastry to the oven and cook for a further 5 minutes until crisp and golden brown. Reduce the oven temperature to 150°C/300°F/Gas 2.

To make the filling, put the cornflour into a pan and add the sugar, lemon rind and 300ml/½ pint/1¼ cups water. Heat the mixture, stirring continuously, until it comes to the boil and thickens. Reduce the heat and simmer very gently for 1 minute. Remove the pan from the heat and stir in the lemon juice.

Add the egg yolks to the lemon mixture, one at a time, beating after each addition, and then stir in the butter. Tip the mixture into the cooled, baked pastry case and level the surface.

To make the topping, whisk the egg whites until stiff peaks form then whisk in half the sugar. Fold in the rest of the sugar using a metal spoon. Spread the meringue over the lemon filling, covering it completely. Cook for about 20 minutes until lightly browned. Serve warm or at room temperature, in slices.

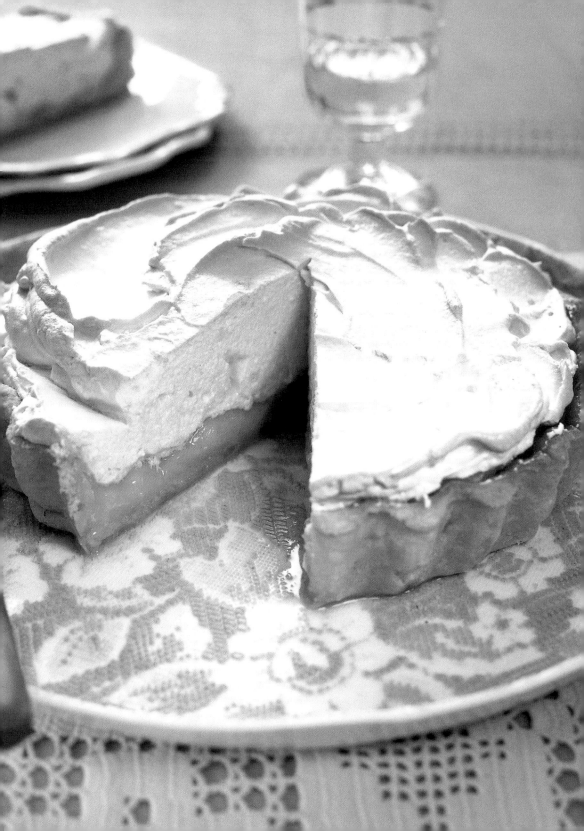

BLUEBERRY AND ALMOND TART

This easy recipe uses the convenience of shop-bought marzipan to add an almondy richness. With its FODMAP-friendly, energizing blueberries, this delightful tart is a classy end to supper. Make sure the marzipan doesn't have added fructose.

Follow the instructions on page 148 and make the pastry the same way as for lemon meringue pie.

Preheat the oven to 200°C/400°F/Gas 6. Roll out the pastry and use to line a 20cm/8in flan tin (pie pan). Line with baking parchment and fill with baking beans, then bake for 15 minutes. Remove the beans and baking parchment and bake for a further 5 minutes. Reduce the oven temperature to 180°C/350°F/Gas 4.

Grate the marzipan. Whisk the egg whites until stiff. Sprinkle half the marzipan over them and fold in. Then fold in the rest.

Turn the mixture into the pastry case (pie shell) and spread it evenly. Sprinkle the blueberries over the top and bake for 20–25 minutes, until golden and just set. Leave to cool for 10 minutes before serving.

FODMAP TYPE: Nil
NUTRITIONAL CONTENT:
Energy 266kcal/1112kJ;
Protein 5g; Carbohydrate 39g,
of which sugars 22g; Fat 11g, of
which saturates 5g; Cholesterol
18mg; Calcium 23mg; Fibre 2g;
Sodium 298mg

Desserts & Baking

SERVES 6

For the pastry
115g/4oz/1 cup wheat-free
    plain (all-purpose) flour
pinch of salt
50g/2oz butter, diced

For the filling
175g/6oz/generous 1 cup white
    fructose-free marzipan
4 large (US extra large) egg
    whites
130g/4½oz/generous 1 cup
    blueberries

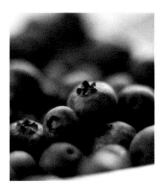

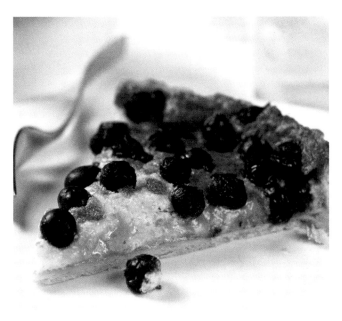

HOT CHOCOLATE SOUFFLÉS

Flour-free, these are the lightest, melt-in-the-mouth soufflés ever, laced with a touch of orange liqueur. They are best made just before serving. If more indulgence is required, serve with Greek yogurt or lactose-free ice cream.

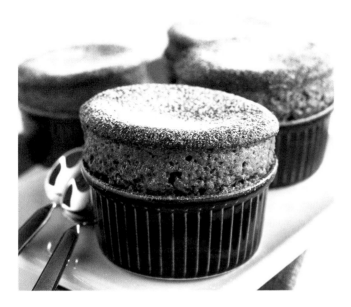

FODMAP TYPE: Lactose
NUTRITIONAL CONTENT:
Energy 569kcal/2388kJ;
Protein 16g; Carbohydrate 67g,
of which sugars 20g; Fat 28g, of
which saturates 2g; Cholesterol
0mg; Calcium 101mg; Fibre 7g;
Sodium 31mg

SERVES 6

butter, for greasing
45ml/3 tbsp caster (superfine)
  sugar, plus extra for dusting
175g/6oz plain (semisweet)
  chocolate, chopped
150g/5oz/²⁄₃ cup unsalted
  butter, cut in small pieces
4 large eggs, separated
30ml/2 tbsp orange liqueur
  (optional)
1.5ml/¼ tsp cream of tartar
icing (confectioners') sugar,
  for dusting

Butter six 150ml/¼ pint/²⁄₃ cup ramekins. Sprinkle each with a little caster sugar and tap out any excess.

Melt the chocolate and butter in a pan on a low heat, stirring occasionally. Remove from the heat and cool slightly, then beat in the egg yolks and orange liqueur, if using. Set aside.

Preheat the oven to 220°C/425°F/Gas 7. In a large bowl, whisk the egg whites until frothy. Add the cream of tartar and whisk until soft peaks form. Gradually sprinkle over the caster sugar, 15ml/1 tbsp at a time, whisking until stiff and glossy.

Stir a third of the whites into the cooled chocolate mixture to lighten it, then fold in the remaining whites with a metal spoon. Spoon into the prepared dishes.

Bake the soufflés for 10–12 minutes until risen and set, but still slightly wobbly in the centre. Dust with icing sugar and serve.

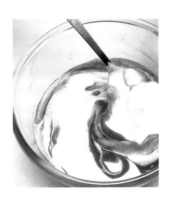

Desserts & Baking

RHUBARB CRUMBLE

Crumble is another classic pudding that can be made low-FODMAP friendly. When rhubarb is out of season, try raspberries or blueberries. Make sure the redcurrant jelly doesn't contain any fructose syrup.

FODMAP TYPE: Nil
NUTRITIONAL CONTENT:
Energy 449kcal/1877kJ;
Protein 7g; Carbohydrate 69g,
of which sugars 32g; Fat 18g, of
which saturates 10g; Cholesterol
40mg; Calcium 129mg; Fibre 6g;
Sodium 139mg

Cook the rhubarb with the sugar, redcurrant jelly and water and until soft but not still holding its shape. Transfer to a deep pie dish. Preheat the oven to 200°C/400°F/Gas 6.

Combine all the ingredients for the topping with your fingers, rubbing in the butter until the mixture has a crumb-like texture. Sprinkle the crumble topping evenly over the fruit.

Bake the crumble at the top of the preheated oven for 20 minutes, or until the top is crunchy and slightly brown. Serve warm with double cream.

Desserts & Baking

SERVES 4

450g/1lb rhubarb
50g/2oz/¼ cup caster
  (superfine) sugar
30ml/2 tbsp redcurrant jelly
45–60ml/3–4 tbsp water
double (heavy) cream, to serve

For the topping
115g/4oz/1 cup buckwheat
  flour
50g/2oz/½ cup oats
50g/2oz/½ cup medium polenta
50g/2oz/¼ cup sugar
75g/3oz butter

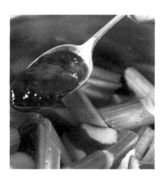

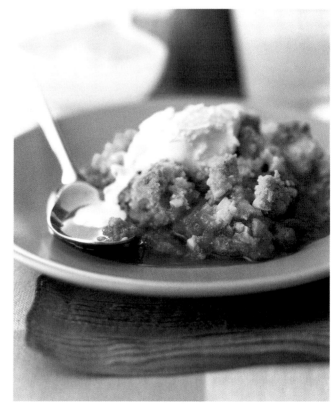

RICE PUDDING WITH ORANGES AND CINNAMON

Rice pudding is such a nurturing dessert, particularly so in this recipe, which adds nutrient-rich oranges, cinnamon and cream. Coconut milk lends a natural sweetness, but can be substituted for any low-lactose alternative.

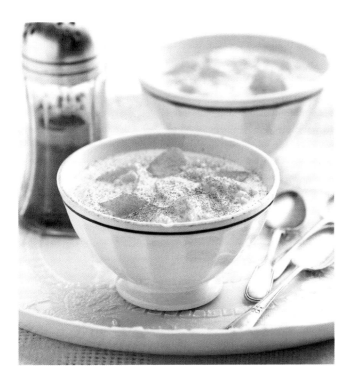

FODMAP TYPE: Polyol (Sorbitol)
NUTRITIONAL CONTENT:
Energy 235kcal/982kJ;
Protein 5g; Carbohydrate 55g,
of which sugars 23g; Fat 1g, of
which saturates 1g; Cholesterol
0mg; Calcium 132mg; Fibre 2g;
Sodium 574mg

SERVES 4

400ml/14fl oz/1⅔ cups water
150g/5oz/¾ cup short grain rice
1 litre/1¾ pints/4 cups coconut
   milk
5ml/1 tsp salt
sugar, to taste
5ml/1 tsp vanilla extract
5ml/1 tsp ground cinnamon,
   plus extra for dusting
2–3 fresh oranges, peeled

Bring the water in a pan to the boil, then slowly add the rice so that the water continues to boil. Reduce the heat and simmer for 10–15 minutes until the water is absorbed.

Add the milk to the rice, return to the boil then simmer for 30–40 minutes until the rice is cooked. Season with the salt and sweeten to taste with the sugar. Add the vanilla extract and cinnamon. Turn into a bowl and leave to cool.

Segment the oranges, cutting down between each piece and its membrane to release and lift out. Cut each segment into three. Fold most of the orange pieces into the rice pudding. Serve at room temperature in little dishes, topped with cinnamon and orange pieces.

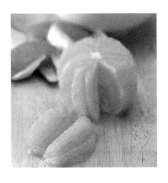

GOAT'S CHEESE CHEESECAKE WITH RASPBERRY SAUCE

With a quirky goat's cheese base, these elegant little baked cheesecakes aren't too sweet. Prettily served bathed in their own wonderful raspberry coulis, they are perfect for advance preparation, and impressing your guests.

FODMAP TYPE: Lactose
NUTRITIONAL CONTENT:
Energy 265kcal/1108kJ;
Protein 9g; Carbohydrate 21g,
of which sugars 21g; Fat 17g, of
which saturates 10g; Cholesterol
120mg; Calcium 122mg; Fibre
4g; Sodium 221mg

Desserts & Baking

SERVES 6

butter, for greasing
225g/8oz/1 cup creamy, thick
    goat's cheese
75g/3oz/⅓ cup soft light brown
    sugar
3 eggs, lightly beaten
120ml/4fl oz/½ cup crème
    fraîche
400g/14oz/2⅓ cups raspberries
30ml/2 tbsp caster (superfine)
    sugar

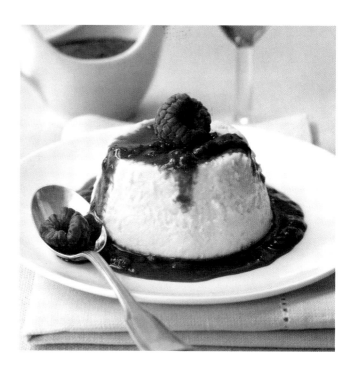

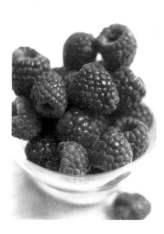

Preheat the oven to 180°C/350°F/Gas 4. Butter six ramekin dishes. Put the goat's cheese and sugar in a bowl and whisk together until light and fluffy. Gradually add the beaten eggs and continue whisking. The mixture will be fairly liquid. Add the crème fraîche and beat for 1 more minute.

Pour the mixture into the ramekin dishes, and put into a roasting pan. Half-fill the pan with warm water, then cook in the oven for 10 minutes. Turn off the oven, leaving the cheesecakes inside for 1 hour to cool slowly.

Meanwhile, put most of the raspberries in a pan with the sugar and cook over a medium heat for 3–5 minutes, or until slightly thickened. Cool. Turn out each cheesecake and serve topped with the sauce and one of the reserved raspberries.

BAKED BANANAS WITH TOFFEE SAUCE

Warm, sweet bananas, baked in their own skins, may induce nostalgic memories of camping out, but you probably wouldn't have been lucky enough to have them doused in toffee sauce.

Preheat the oven to 180°C/350°F/Gas 4. Put the unpeeled bananas in an ovenproof dish and bake for 15–20 minutes, until the skins are very dark and the flesh feels soft when pushed slightly.

Meanwhile, heat the light muscovado sugar in a small, heavy pan with 75ml/5 tbsp water until dissolved. Bring to the boil and add the double cream. Cook for 5 minutes, until the sauce has thickened and is toffee-coloured. Remove from the heat.

Transfer the baked bananas in their skins to serving plates and split them lengthways to reveal the flesh. Drizzle a little toffee sauce over the bananas and serve, together with some lactose-free or soya ice cream, if you wish.

FODMAP TYPE: Lactose
NUTRITIONAL CONTENT:
Energy 255kcal/1066kJ;
Protein 2g; Carbohydrate 42g,
of which sugars 40g; Fat 10g, of
which saturates 6g; Cholesterol
26mg; Calcium 26mg; Fibre 3g;
Sodium 11mg

SERVES 4

4 large bananas
75g/3oz/scant ½ cup light
    muscovado (brown) sugar
75ml/5 tbsp double (heavy)
    cream
lactose-free or soya ice cream,
    to serve (optional)

Desserts & Baking

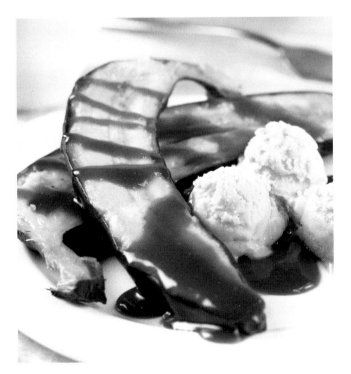

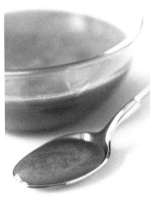

PANNA COTTA

This Italian classic traditionally used egg whites to thicken the cream, often left over after the yolks had been used to enrich pasta or pastries. Now, however, gelatine is more often used to set these delicate little desserts.

FODMAP TYPE: Lactose
NUTRITIONAL CONTENT:
Energy 297kcal/1241kJ;
Protein 5g; Carbohydrate 17g,
of which sugars 17g; Fat 24g, of
which saturates 15g; Cholesterol
68mg; Calcium 119mg; Fibre 0g;
Sodium 43mg

SERVES 8

1 litre/1¾ pints/4 cups single
(light) cream
50g/2oz/½ cup icing
(confectioners') sugar
3 or 4 sheets gelatine
60ml/4 tbsp caster (superfine)
sugar

VARIATIONS You can add flavourings if you like, such as coffee, vanilla extract, crushed berries or a dash of liqueur.

Divide the single cream in half and put it into two separate pans. Bring the cream in both pans to just under the boil over a low-medium heat. To one pan of cream add the icing sugar, and to the other add the sheets of gelatine.

Whisk the cream in both pans constantly until the sugar and gelatine have completely dissolved and the cream is very hot but not boiling.

Pour the cream from both pans into one bowl and whisk together. Allow the mixture to cool completely.

While the mixture is cooling, put the caster sugar into a small pan and melt over a low heat without stirring until caramelized to a light blond colour.

Coat the base of eight small metal moulds or ramekins with the caramel. Allow the caramel to cool.

Strain the cooled panna cotta into the moulds and put into the refrigerator to set. When firmly set, dip the moulds into boiling water for 5 seconds and turn out on to cold plates.

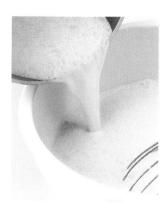
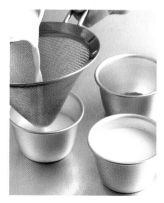

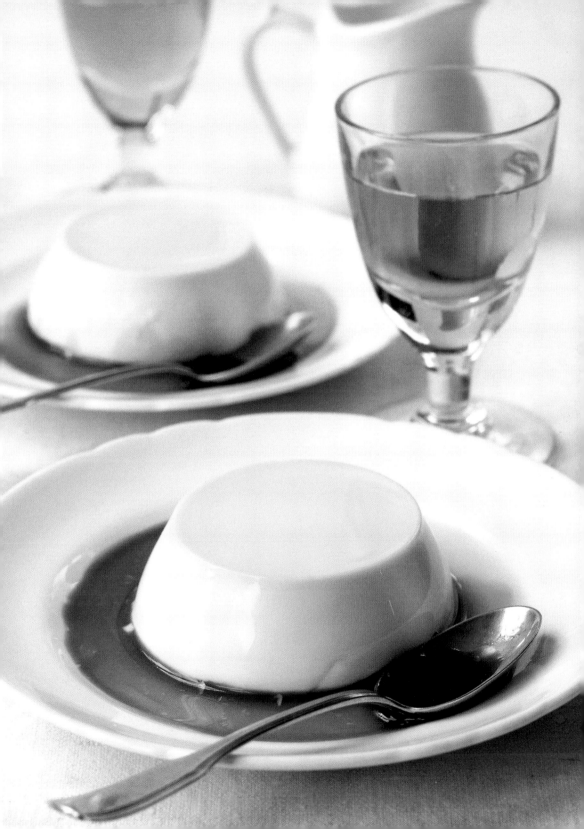

RHUBARB COMPOTE

Scandinavians love fruit served this way, and will eat their 'sweet soups' either warm or cold, as part of a main meal or for breakfast. Don't be shy of potato flour, which is a low-FODMAP flour that will thicken instantly with hot water.

Desserts & Baking

FODMAP TYPE: Lactose
NUTRITIONAL CONTENT:
Energy 165kcal/6 kJ; Protein 2g;
Carbohydrate 44g, of which
sugars 39g; Fat 0g, of which
saturates 0g; Cholesterol 0mg;
Calcium 138mg; Fibre 3g;
Sodium 213mg

SERVES 4

500g/1¼lb rhubarb, cut into
    small lengths
1 cinnamon stick (optional)
150g/5oz/¾ cup sugar
25g/1oz potato flour
pinch of salt
crème fraîche, to serve

VARIATIONS Use the same quantity of strawberries and add a small piece of fresh root ginger, grated.

In a pan, bring 1.2 litre/2 pints/5 cups of water to the boil. Add the rhubarb and cinnamon stick and simmer for about 5 minutes, until the rhubarb is soft. Remove the cinnamon and add sugar to taste.

Put the potato flour in a small bowl, add a little water and blend together to form a smooth paste. Add to the rhubarb and heat, stirring all the time, until thickened and clear, but do not bring to the boil. Remove from the heat and add the salt.

Serve the compote hot or cold and garnish each bowl with a spoonful of crème fraîche.

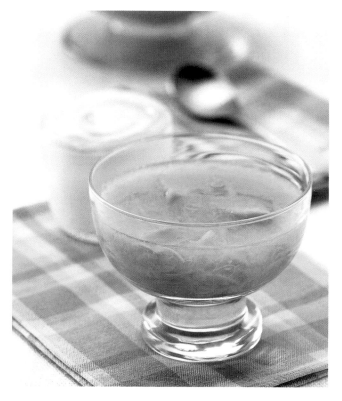

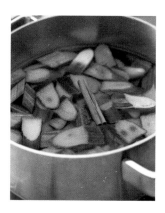

ORANGE JELLY

The recipe for this beautiful jelly comes from Sicily, which is why it is flavoured with the famous Italian liqueur, Limoncello. This jelly is also delicious made from clementine juice too, just substitute the same amount.

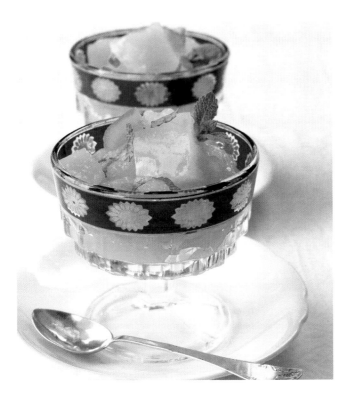

FODMAP TYPE: Fructose
NUTRITIONAL CONTENT:
Energy 75kcal/314kJ;
Protein 3g; Carbohydrate 17g,
of which sugars 17g; Fat 0g, of
which saturates 0g; Cholesterol
0mg; Calcium 26mg; Fibre 0g;
Sodium 21mg

SERVES 6

600ml/20fl oz/2½ cups freshly
   squeezed orange juice
10 sheets leaf gelatine
50g/2oz/¼ cup sugar
handful of fresh mint leaves,
   chopped
Limoncello liqueur,
   for drizzling

Desserts & Baking

Put the orange juice in a pan with 150ml/¼ pint/⅔ cup water. Soak the gelatine in a small bowl of cold water for 5 minutes or until floppy, then drain, squeeze and add it to the pan.

Add the sugar to the pan. Stir vigorously over a low heat until the sugar has dissolved and the gelatine has melted completely.

Pour into a shallow square or rectangular mould. Chill until firm. Remove the set jelly from the refrigerator, and cut into rough cubes.

Arrange in four stemmed glasses, scatter with the mint leaves and drizzle with Limoncello.

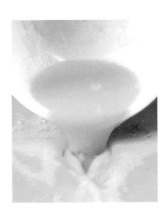

PINEAPPLE AND SPICED FRUIT GRANITAS

Containing tropical papaya, pineapple and orange juice, but in sufficiently dilute quantities, this a refreshing iced treat with contrasting grilled fruit. Granitas are not stirred so frequently during freezing as sorbets, giving a coarser texture.

FODMAP TYPE: Fructose
NUTRITIONAL CONTENT:
Energy 512kcal/2140kJ;
Protein 4g; Carbohydrate 134g,
of which sugars 129g; Fat 1g, of
which saturates 0g; Cholesterol
0mg; Calcium 110mg; Fibre 3g;
Sodium 46mg

Desserts & Baking

SERVES 8

1 small pineapple
2 bananas
45–60ml/3–4 tbsp icing
(confectioners') sugar

For the papaya granita
4 papayas, peeled, deseeded
and diced
250g/9oz/1¼ cups caster
(superfine) sugar
juice of ½ lemon
15ml/1 tbsp orange flower
water
2.5ml/½ tsp ground cinnamon

For the spiced orange granita
900ml/1½ pints/3¾ cups water
350g/12oz/1¾ cups sugar
5–6 cloves
5ml/1 tsp ground ginger
2.5ml/½ tsp ground cinnamon
600ml/1 pint/2½ cups orange
juice
15ml/1 tbsp orange flower
water

To make the papaya granita, purée the papaya flesh in a blender. Put the sugar with 150ml/¼ pint/⅔ cup water in a pan and stir until dissolved. Bring to the boil, simmer for 5 minutes, then set aside to cool.

Stir in the lemon juice, orange flower water and cinnamon, then beat in the papaya purée. Pour the mixture into a bowl; place in the freezer. Stir every 15 minutes for 2 hours and then at intervals for 1 hour, so that the mixture freezes but is slushy.

To make the spiced orange granita, heat the water and sugar together in a pan with the cloves, stirring until the sugar has dissolved, then bring to the boil and boil for about 5 minutes. Leave to cool and stir in the ginger, cinnamon, orange juice and orange flower water.

Remove the cloves, then pour the mixture into a bowl, cover and place in the freezer. Freeze as for the papaya granita.

Just before serving, peel, core and slice the pineapple, and peel and halve the bananas.

Preheat the grill (broiler) on the hottest setting. Arrange the fruit on a baking sheet. Sprinkle with icing sugar and grill for 3–4 minutes until slightly softened and lightly browned.

Arrange the fruit on a serving platter and scoop the granitas into little glasses. Serve immediately.

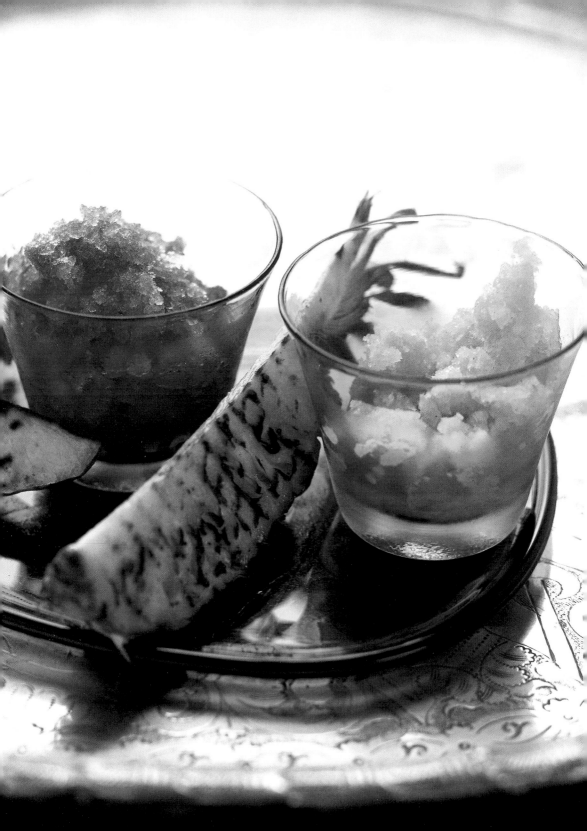

BLUEBERRY ICE CREAM PARFAIT

Of French origin, parfait is a frozen blend of cream, sugar and eggs, like ice cream, but easier, as there is no stirring needed as it freezes. Served here in a terrine-shaped block, you could also have fun with moulds.

FODMAP TYPE: Lactose
NUTRITIONAL CONTENT:
Energy 371kcal/1551kJ;
Protein 4g; Carbohydrate 26g,
of which sugars 24g; Fat 29g of
which saturates 17g; Cholesterol
146mg; Calcium 38mg; Fibre 1g;
Sodium 41mg

Desserts & Baking

SERVES 6

2 large eggs, separated
115g/4oz/1 cup icing
    (confectioners') sugar
200g/7oz/1¾ cup blueberries
300ml/½ pint/1¼ cups double
    (heavy) cream
30ml/2 tbsp aquavit (optional)

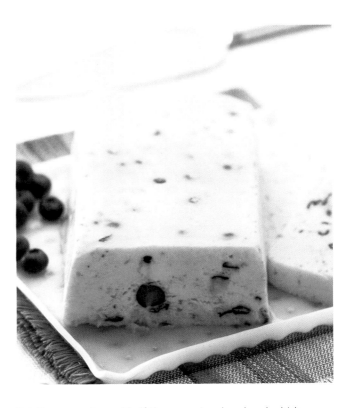

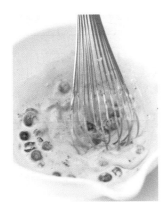

Put the egg yolks and half the sugar in a bowl and whisk together until pale and thick. Beat in about three-quarters of the blueberries and reserve the remainder for decorating. Blend in the berries so that they burst and spread their colour.

Whisk the egg whites until they stand in soft peaks, then whisk in the remaining sugar. Fold into the blueberry mixture. Whisk the cream with the aquavit, if using, until it just holds its shape, and fold into the blueberry mixture. Transfer to a mould or freezer container and freeze for 6–8 hours until firm.

To serve, dip the mould briefly in hot water before turning out, decorate with the reserved blueberries and cut into slices.

COCONUT MILK AND LIME ICE CREAM

The flesh of coconut contains FODMAP sorbitol, which is also used in low-calorie sweeteners. In coconut milk, however, this is sufficiently diluted, which makes it a handy addition to both sweet and savoury foods.

Put the water and sugar in a small pan and bring to the boil, stirring constantly until the sugar has dissolved. Remove the pan from the heat and leave the syrup to cool, then chill well.

Grate the limes, taking care to avoid the bitter pith. Squeeze them and pour the juice and rind into the pan of syrup. Add the coconut milk.

Pour the mixture into a plastic tub and freeze for 5–6 hours until firm, beating twice with a fork, electric whisk or in a food processor to break up the crystals. Scoop into dishes and decorate with toasted coconut shavings.

FODMAP TYPE: Polyol (Sorbitol)
NUTRITIONAL CONTENT:
Energy 126kcal/527kJ;
Protein Trace; Carbohydrate
34g, of which sugars 34g;
Fat Trace; Cholesterol 0mg;
Calcium 46mg; Fibre 0g;
Sodium 118mg

SERVES 4

163

150ml/¼ pint/⅔ cup water
115g/4oz/½ cup caster
   (superfine) sugar
2 limes
400ml/14fl oz can coconut milk
toasted coconut shavings,
   to decorate

Desserts & Baking

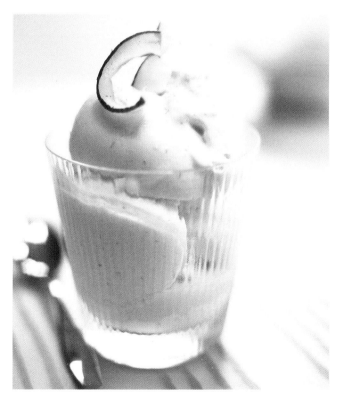

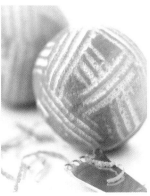

RASPBERRY SHERBET

Traditional sherbets from the Middle East are made in much the same way as sorbets but with added milk. This version is made from raspberry purée blended with sugar syrup and crème fraîche then flecked with crushed raspberries.

FODMAP TYPE: Lactose
NUTRITIONAL CONTENT:
Energy 440kcal/1839kJ;
Protein 3g; Carbohydrate 35g,
of which sugars 35g; Fat 33g, of
which saturates 23g; Cholesterol
93mg; Calcium 85mg; Fibre 6g;
Sodium 30mg

Desserts & Baking

SERVES 6

175g/6oz/¾ cup caster
  (superfine) sugar
150ml/¼ pint/⅔ cup water
500g/1¼lb/3½ cups raspberries,
  plus extra, to serve
500ml/17fl oz/generous 2 cups
  crème fraîche

Put the sugar and water in a small pan and bring to the boil, stirring until the sugar has dissolved. Pour into a bowl and cool.

Put 350g/12oz/2½ cups of the raspberries in a food processor or blender. Process to a purée, then strain over a large bowl to remove the seeds. Stir the sugar syrup into the raspberry purée and chill the mixture until it is very cold.

Add the crème fraîche to the purée and whisk until smooth. Pour the mixture into a plastic tub and freeze for 4 hours, beating once with a fork, electric whisk or in a food processor to break up the ice crystals. After this time, beat it again.

Crush the remaining raspberries between your fingers and fold in to the partially frozen ice cream. Freeze for 2–3 hours until firm. Serve with extra raspberries.

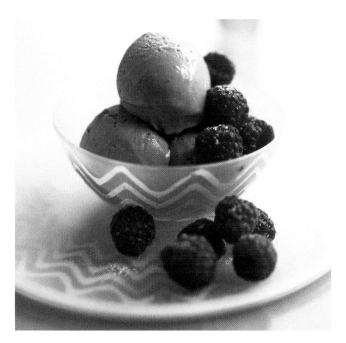

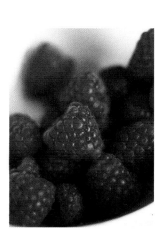

CHOCOLATE ESPRESSO MOUSSE

This classic chocolate mousse is made with good quality dark chocolate that thankfully is FODMAP-free. It could also be served sundae-style, layered in a tall glass with crushed meringues, natural yogurt and sliced bananas.

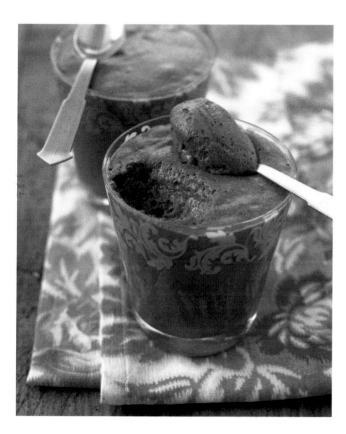

FODMAP TYPE: Lactose
NUTRITIONAL CONTENT:
Energy 370kcal/1547kJ;
Protein 10g; Carbohydrate 52g,
of which sugars 52g; Fat 16g, of
which saturates 7g; Cholesterol
262mg; Calcium 67mg; Fibre 1g;
Sodium 105mg

SERVES 6

Desserts & Baking

175g/6oz dark (bittersweet)
   chocolate (minimum 70 per
   cent cocoa solids)
60ml/4 tbsp cooled strong
   espresso coffee
8 eggs, separated
200g/7oz/1 cup caster
   (superfine) sugar

Break the chocolate into small pieces and melt in a heatproof bowl over a pan of simmering water. Once the chocolate has completely melted, stir in the cold coffee. Leave to cool slightly.

Beat the egg yolks with half the sugar until it is pale, thick and creamy. Stir in the melted chocolate mixture.

Whisk the egg whites in a separate bowl until stiff peaks form. Stir in the remaining sugar, then fold into the chocolate mixture. Spoon into chilled glasses or ramekins and chill for at least 3–4 hours before serving.

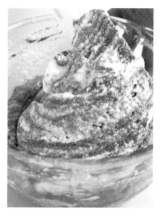

BERRY AND CARDAMOM MERINGUES

These homemade nutty meringues are crisp on the outside, and nicely moistened by the natural nut oils on the inside. Meringues are easy to make, but take care when separating eggs, as any yolk will prevent the whites from foaming.

FODMAP TYPE: GOS
NUTRITIONAL CONTENT:
Energy 527kcal/2203kJ;
Protein 6g; Carbohydrate 51g,
of which sugars 50g; Fat 35g, of
which saturates 13g; Cholesterol
45mg; Calcium 61mg; Fibre 2g;
Sodium 91mg

SERVES 6

1.5ml/¼ tsp cardamom seeds
4 large (US extra large) egg
   whites
250g/9oz/generous 2 cups icing
   (confectioners') sugar
75g/2oz/½ cup ground almonds
75g/2oz/½ cup ground
   macadamia nuts
200ml/7fl oz/scant 1 cup double
   (heavy) cream, whipped
200g/7oz/scant 2 cups fresh
   berries, chopped if large
30ml/2 tbsp fructose-free
   raspberry jam

Preheat the oven to 200°C/400°F/Gas 6 and line two large baking sheets with baking parchment. Grind the cardamom seeds finely using a mortar and pestle.

Put the egg whites into a clean, grease-free bowl and whisk until they form stiff peaks. Using a wooden spoon, slowly and gently fold in the icing sugar a little at a time.

Fold in the ground almonds and macadamia nuts, together with the cardamom. You should have a smooth mixture.

Using a teaspoon, spoon dollops of the mixture on to the baking parchment, about 5cm/2in apart.

Bake for 8–10 minutes, or until golden. Leave the meringues to cool on the sheet.

Combine the cream, berries and raspberry jam, and use the mixture to make little meringue sandwiches.

COOK'S TIP Make your own ground macadamia nuts by blitzing them in a food processor until very fine. Use low-FODMAP berries like raspberries, blueberries or strawberries and avoid blackberries and cherries.

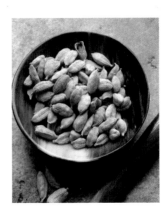
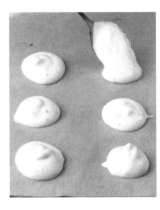

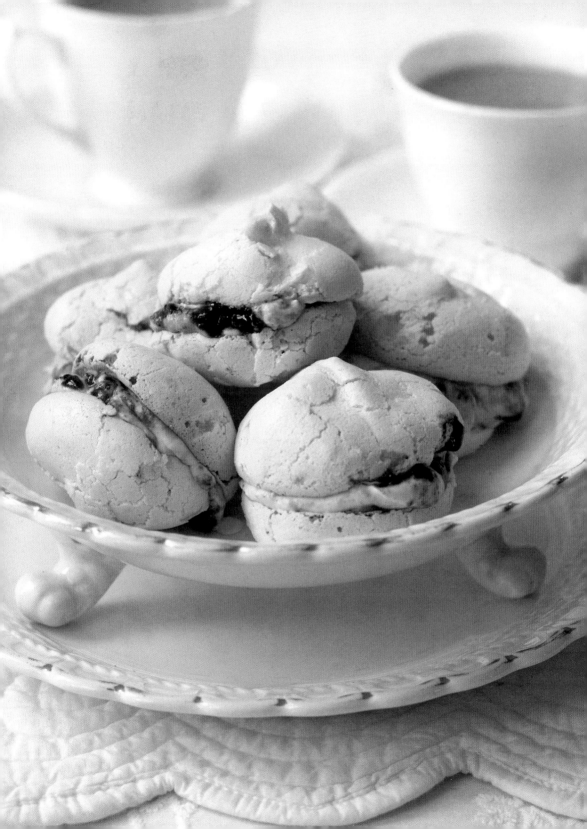

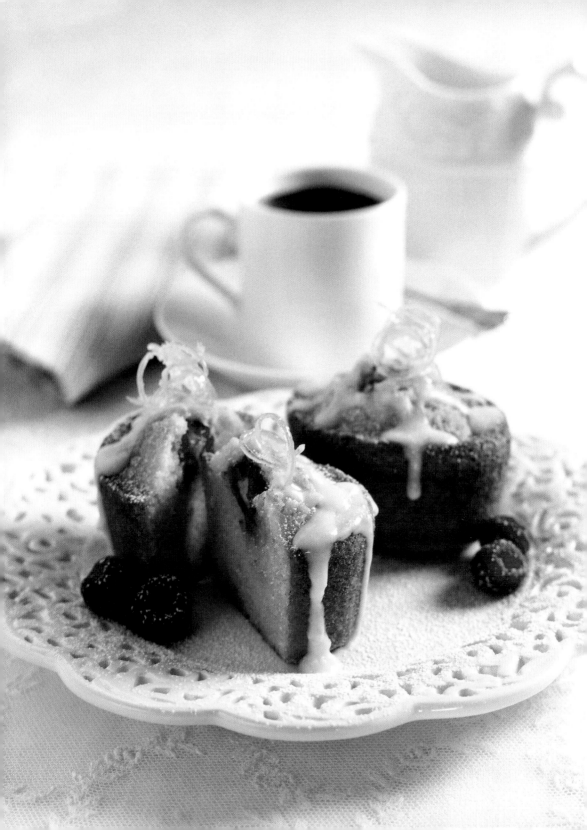

RASPBERRY FRIANDS

Friands are small cakes of French origin that are now popular all over the world. Use any wheat-free flour to your liking or convenience, for example rice or cornflour, which complements the richness of ground almonds.

Preheat the oven to 200°C/400°F/Gas 6. Grease the cups of a friand or bun tin (muffin pan) with melted butter and dust lightly with flour. Turn the tin upside down and tap it sharply on the work surface to get rid of any excess flour.

Melt the butter, remove from the heat and set aside to cool slightly. Put the ground almonds, sugar and flour in a mixing bowl and stir together.

In a separate bowl, beat the egg whites lightly for 15 seconds, or just enough to break them up.

Add the egg whites to the dry ingredients and mix. Add the melted butter to the bowl and mix lightly until just combined.

Pour the mixture into the cups and press one raspberry into the centre of each. Bake for 20–25 minutes until the friands are pale golden and springy to the touch. Leave to cool slightly then turn them out on to a wire rack.

To make the sugar frosting, mix the lemon juice with the sugar and set aside for 10 minutes for the sugar to partly dissolve.

Drizzle the icing over the tops of the cooled cakes and leave to set until set. Top with a few curls of candied lemon rind and a dusting of icing sugar, and serve with a few fresh raspberries.

FODMAP TYPE: GOS
NUTRITIONAL CONTENT:
Energy 309kcal/1292kJ;
Protein 3g; Carbohydrate 38g,
of which sugars 33g; Fat 18g, of
which saturates 8g; Cholesterol
31mg; Calcium 35mg; Fibre 1g;
Sodium 98mg

MAKES 12

175g/6oz/¾ cup butter
115g/4oz/1 cup ground
  almonds
225g/8oz/2 cups icing
  (confectioners') sugar, sifted,
  plus extra for dusting
70g/2½oz/9 tbsp plain
  (all-purpose) wheat-free
  flour, sifted
6 egg whites
115g/4oz/¾ cup fresh
  raspberries

For the crunchy sugar frosting
juice of 1 small lemon
150g/5oz/¾ cup caster
  (superfine) sugar
very finely cut strips of candied
  lemon rind

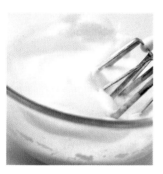
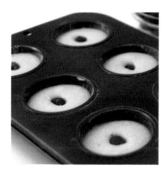

POLENTA CAKE

Polenta is a golden-yellow cornmeal made from dried, ground maize (corn), and is popular as an Italian store cupboard staple. This is a crumbly cake, with a rich, granular texture, perfect as a morning coffee accompaniment.

FODMAP TYPE: GOS
NUTRITIONAL CONTENT:
Energy 388kcal/1622kJ;
Protein 7g; Carbohydrate 68g,
of which sugars 39g; Fat 12g, of
which saturates 3g; Cholesterol
131mg; Calcium 68mg; Fibre 3g;
Sodium 182mg

SERVES 8

75g/3oz/⅔ cup blanched
   almonds
300g/11oz/generous 1½ cups
   sugar
300g/11oz/2¾ cups fine yellow
   polenta
grated rind of 1 lemon
3 egg yolks
90ml/6 tbsp single (light) cream
pinch of salt
butter, for greasing
flaked (sliced) almonds,
   to decorate

Preheat the oven to 180°C/350°F/Gas 4. Butter a shallow 20cm/8in cake tin (pan) well.

Grind the almonds finely using a mortar and pestle or in a food processor, then mix them with the sugar, polenta and the lemon rind in a large bowl.

Mix in the egg yolks and the cream to make a thick but wet dough. Stir in a pinch of salt. Pour into the cake tin and bake for 20 minutes, until firm and crisp. Cool in the tin, then sprinkle with flaked almonds and serve with coffee or hot chocolate, if you like.

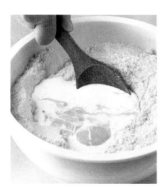

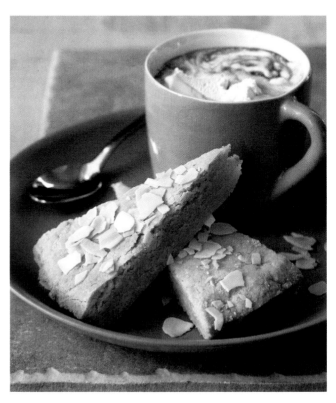

ITALIAN RICE CAKE

This carbohydrate-rich cake, a kind of baked rice pudding, is a delicious coffee-time treat, or serve it as a dessert with fresh clementines or low-FODMAP berries. Use more lemon or lime zest for a sharper flavour.

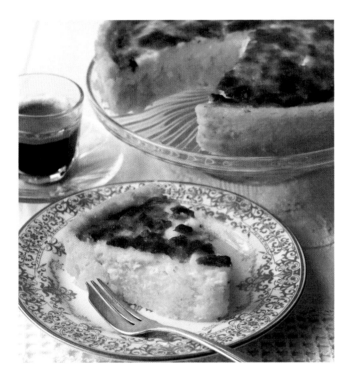

FODMAP TYPE: Nil
NUTRITIONAL CONTENT:
Energy 314kcal/1313kJ;
Protein 13g; Carbohydrate 46g,
of which sugars 30g; Fat 9g, of
which saturates 2g; Cholesterol
219mg; Calcium 68mg; Fibre
Trace; Sodium 136mg

SERVES

Desserts & Baking

150g/5oz/⅔ cup short grain rice
1.2 litres/2 pints/5 cups rice milk
butter, for greasing
9 eggs
225g/8oz/generous 1 cup caster
    (superfine) sugar
45ml/3 tbsp brandy
grated rind of 1 unwaxed
    lemon

Put the rice and 750ml/1¼ pints/3 cups of the milk into a pan. Boil for 10 minutes, then drain, reserving the milk, which will have absorbed some of the starch from the rice. Set aside to cool. Preheat the oven to 180°C/350°F/Gas 4.

Butter a 25cm/10in fixed-base cake tin (pan). Using an electric whisk, beat the eggs in a large bowl until foaming and pale yellow. Add the sugar gradually, beating constantly, then add the brandy and lemon rind. Stir well.

Add the rice and remaining milk (including the reserved milk). Pour into the cake tin. Bake for 50 minutes, or until a cocktail stick (toothpick) inserted into the centre comes out clean. The cake should be well set and golden brown. Serve warm or cold.

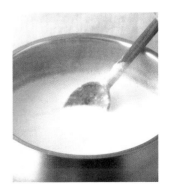

COURGETTE AND GINGER CAKE

Like carrot or beetroot, courgette adds an unexpected moistness to baking, particularly with oil used in the place of butter. A lovely teatime or lunch box stand-by this cake slices easily and is delicious spread generously with butter.

FODMAP TYPE: Nil
NUTRITIONAL CONTENT:
Energy 426kcal/1781kJ;
Protein 4g; Carbohydrate 54g,
of which sugars 25g; Fat 23g, of
which saturates 4g; Cholesterol
59mg; Calcium 28mg; Fibre 1g;
Sodium 49mg

Desserts & Baking

SERVES 8–10

3 eggs
225g/8oz/generous 1 cup caster
  (superfine) sugar
250ml/8fl oz/1 cup sunflower oil
5ml/1 tsp vanilla extract
15ml/1 tbsp syrup from a jar of
  stem ginger
225g/8oz courgettes (zucchini),
  grated
2.5cm/1in piece fresh root
  ginger, grated
115g/4oz/1 cup each of potato
  flour, tapioca flour, maize
  flour and buckwheat flour
5ml/1 tsp baking powder
pinch of salt
5ml/1 tsp ground cinnamon
2 pieces stem ginger, chopped
15ml/1 tbsp demerara (raw)
  sugar

VARIATION Spoon the mixture into muffin cases to make individual little cakes, if you wish.

Preheat the oven to 190°C/325°F/Gas 5. Beat together the eggs and sugar until light and fluffy. Slowly beat in the oil until the mixture forms a batter. Mix in the vanilla extract and ginger syrup, then stir in the courgettes and fresh ginger.

Sift together the flours, baking powder and salt into a large bowl. Add the cinnamon and mix well, then stir the dried ingredients into the courgette mixture.

Line a 900g/2lb loaf tin (pan) with baking parchment and pour in the cake mixture. Smooth and level the top, then sprinkle the chopped stem ginger and demerara sugar over the surface.

Bake for 1 hour until a skewer inserted into the centre comes out clean. Leave the cake in the tin to cool for about 20 minutes, then turn out on to a wire rack.

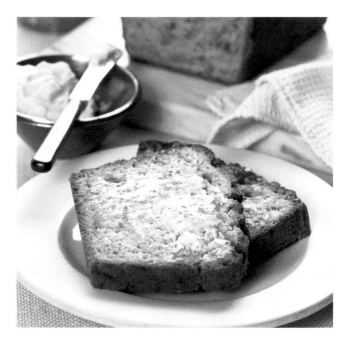

RICE, BUCKWHEAT AND CORN BREAD

Replicating the lightness of regular flour can be a challenge in wheat-free baking, but this loaf uses a blend of rustic flours and a generous amount of yeast and sugar to give a good rise, and makes for an excellent open-textured loaf.

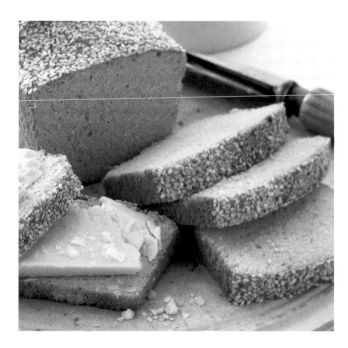

FODMAP TYPE: Lactose
NUTRITIONAL CONTENT:
Energy 191kcal/798kJ;
Protein 4g; Carbohydrate 30g,
of which sugars 1g; Fat 5g, of
which saturates 2g; Cholesterol
24mg; Calcium 47mg; Fibre 3g;
Sodium 200mg

SERVES 12

173

Desserts & Baking

200ml/7fl oz/scant 1 cup tepid
 semi-skimmed (low-fat) milk
200ml/7fl oz/scant 1 cup tepid
 water
350g/12oz/3 cups brown
 rice flour
50g/2oz/½ cup buckwheat flour
 or soya flour
50g/2oz/½ cup gluten-free
 cornmeal
5ml/1 tsp caster (superfine)
 sugar
5ml/1 tsp salt
7g/¼oz sachet easy-blend
 (rapid-rise) dried yeast
40g/1½oz/3 tbsp soft butter
1 medium egg, beaten, plus
 extra for glazing
30ml/2 tbsp sesame seeds

Lightly grease a 900g/2lb loaf tin (pan). Mix the milk and water together in a measuring jug or cup.

Place the rice flour, buckwheat or soya flour, cornmeal, sugar and salt in a bowl and stir in the dried yeast. Lightly rub in the butter until the mixture resembles fine breadcrumbs.

Add the milk and water mixture and the egg and beat together to form a smooth, thick consistency. Spoon into the prepared tin, then cover and leave in a warm place until it has risen to the top of the tin. Preheat the oven to 200°C/400°F/Gas 6.

Brush the top of the bread with a little beaten egg and scatter the sesame seeds over it. Bake for 30 minutes until lightly browned. Turn out on to a wire rack to cool slightly, and serve warm, sliced and spread with butter or topped with cheese.

INDEX

Index

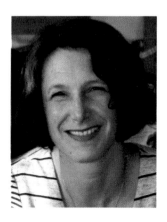

PENNY DOYLE is an inspired food writer and cook, who is also a qualified and highly experienced dietitian and nutritional consultant. A specialist in coeliac disease, irritable bowel syndrome and diabetes, she has recently completed a specialist FODMAP training course, and maintains a keen interest in monitoring research developments. She has extensive clinical experience from both her National Health Service work as a dietitian and her own freelance consultancy. Penny's passion for balanced and delicious food is underpinned by her wide knowledge and experience of healthy eating. Please see her website, www.nutrisult.com, for more information.

Acknowledgements

This edition is published by Lorenz Books, an imprint of Anness Publishing Ltd, 108 Great Russell Street, London WC1B 3NA; info@anness.com; www.lorenzbooks.com; www.annesspublishing.com; twitter: @Anness_Books

If you like the images in this book and would like to investigate using them for publishing, promotions or advertising, please visit our website www.practicalpictures.com for more information.

© Anness Publishing Ltd 2015

All rights reserved. No part of this publication may be reproduced, stored in a retrieval system, or transmitted in any way or by any means, electronic, mechanical, photocopying, recording or otherwise, without the prior written permission of the copyright holder.

A CIP catalogue record for this book is available from the British Library.

Publisher: Joanna Lorenz, Project Editor: Joanne Rippin
Designer: Adelle Mahoney

PUBLISHER'S NOTE
This book provides information on health and medical matters, but is not intended as a substitute for professional diagnosis. Any person with a condition or symptoms requiring medical attention should consult a doctor or fully qualified practitioner. Although the advice and information in this book are believed to be accurate and true at the time of going to press, neither the authors nor the publisher can accept any legal responsibility or liability for any errors or omissions that may have been made nor for any inaccuracies nor for any loss, harm or injury that comes about from following instructions or advice in this book.

COOK'S NOTES
Bracketed terms are intended for American readers.
For all recipes, quantities are given in both metric and imperial measures and, where appropriate, in standard cups and spoons. Follow one set of measures, but not a mixture, as they are not interchangeable.
Standard spoon and cup measures are level. 1 tsp = 5ml, 1 tbsp = 15ml, 1 cup = 250ml/8fl oz.
Australian standard tablespoons are 20ml. Australian readers should use 3 tsp in place of 1 tbsp for measuring small quantities.
American pints are 16fl oz/2 cups. American readers should use 20fl oz/2.5 cups in place of 1 pint when measuring liquids.
Electric oven temperatures in this book are for conventional ovens. When using a fan oven, the temperature will probably need to be reduced by about 10–20°C/20–40°F. Since ovens vary, you should check with your manufacturer's instruction book for guidance.
The nutritional analysis given for each recipe is calculated per portion (i.e. serving or item), unless otherwise stated.
If the recipe gives a range, such as Serves 4–6, then the nutritional analysis will be for the smaller portion size, i.e. 6 servings. The analysis does not include optional ingredients, such as salt added to taste.
Medium (US large) eggs are used unless otherwise stated.

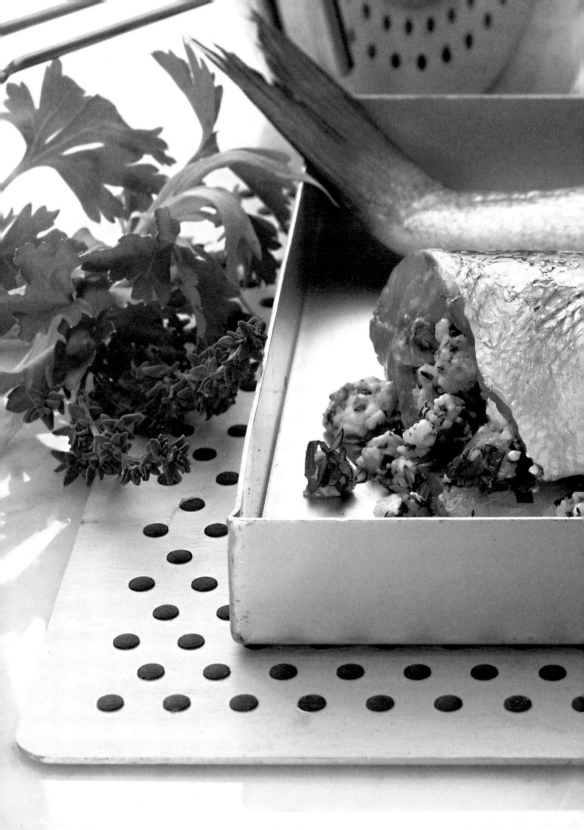